BIRTH AT HOME

Birth at Home

Twenty-one women and their doctor share their experiences of birth

Dr David Miller D. Obst. R.C.O.G. (Lon.)

Photographs by John McCormick

DOUBLEDAY
Sydney   Auckland   New York   Toronto   London

Acknowledgments

Lots of people have contributed in various ways. As well as those who have contributed their stories I want to thank Susie Eisenhuth for showing me how to write what I am trying to say; my friends, Stephen Wall, Stuart Fox, Frank Hall, and my sister, Kathy Golski for badgering me into continuing when I felt like giving up; to Nean Miller, Gayle Cotterell and Therese Holland who skillfully typed into shape my defiant manuscript, as well as my secretaries Jane Haines and Liz Jackson for holding the fort, and soothing the sick and needy while I ran off to births.

To Jude Holland and Pam Sonia my team-mates, who you will get to know through the stories, and who have been constant sources of strength and inspiration.

First published in Australasia in 1990 by Doubleday, a division of Transworld Publishers (Aust.) Pty Limited
15-25 Helles Avenue, Moorebank NSW 2170

Text copyright © David Miller
Photography copyright © John McCormick

All rights reserved. No part of this publication may be reproduced, stored in a retrieval system, transmitted in any form or by any means, electronic, mechanical, photocopying, recording or otherwise, without the prior permission of the publishers.

National Library of Australia
Cataloguing-in-Publication data

Miller, David, 1946 Jan 12-
    Birth at home.

    ISBN 0 86824 422 8.

    1. Childbirth at home - Case studies.
    2. Underwater childbirth - Case studies.
    I. Title.

618.4

Designed by Steven Dunbar
Set in New Caledonia
Printed in Singapore by Kyodo Printing Co Ltd

Preface

Thank you to all the people whose labours have contributed to this book. I'm grateful to them for so honestly describing their experiences for the benefit of other women and families.

Just as a man can never really feel what it is like to labour, so also for a woman who has never delivered a baby. Even for those who have been there, the memory seems often distorted or even totally expunged, so powerful or painful was the experience. For those fortunate enough to have conscious childbirth, the memory is often expressed as life's greatest experience.

I hope these stories are an inspiration and a guide to the positive experience of labour and the enormous fulfilling satisfaction of having laboured and delivered a child.

There is no doubt that labour is often very hard and I am full of admiration for the women I have witnessed at this task. Sometimes even the most careful preparation and hard labour is frustrated by some obstetrical complication which makes surgical or medical intervention necessary, and this needs to be accepted without a sense of failure or feelings of self-doubt. After all, we are lucky to live in an age with the scientific and technical facilities to save life. How we use it, is the issue.

There is no doubt that it is better to have laboured and lost than never to have laboured at all. Women who deliver by 'cold' caesarian section (without labour) sometimes express a feeling of difficulty in bonding, as though there is a missing connection with the child.

I do not think I have ever heard these sentiments from a woman who has worked in labour.

Dedicated to my children Jake and Leah

Contents

Foreword 8
Introduction 11
Looking Back — A Country Doctor's Personal Journey 15

The Stories

Home Births
My First Home Birth: To Graham and Sylvia a son, Billie 59
Elsbeth's Baby: Home Birth After Caesarian 62
Violet: Born in the Garden. Why Not? 67
Lani Joy: A Grandmother's Story 70
Daniel: Boy in a Hurry 79
Baby Cassie: Born on a Mountain 82
A First Baby for Chris: Full Moon Rising 87

The Water Birth Alternative
Mereki: My First Water Birth 93
Birth in the Hidden Valley 97
Nisa: A Family Birth Outdoors 103
Shirley and the Seven Babies: Birth on a Bus! 107
Albie: The Almost-finished Home Birth 112
Yaan: Water Birth by the Ocean 114
Isaan-Julian: A Supportive Second Birth 117
Alana: A Midwife Delivers Her Daughter 119
Pam's Benjamin: The Team Reverses Roles 124

Difficult Situations
Jenny: Breech at Home 134
Off to Hospital 137
Kristie: Exhaustion After Childbirth 142
Margaret: Loss of a Daughter 148
Flood Rescue Baby: Tina's Story 151

Comparative Home Birth Statistics 158

Foreword

This book by Dr David Miller will make the Byron shire of northern New South Wales a focal point for the new consciousness about childbirth.

We already know about Holland where one baby out of three is born at home. But culturally Europe is still made up of compartments with impenetrable barriers: the Dutch example cannot easily spread.

Things are different in the Byron shire. Of course it is a tiny spot compared to Holland. But while home birth is an established institution in Holland, in New South Wales it is still moving towards acceptance. This shift is likely to continue in other places. During a recent lecturing tour, I felt that the collective awareness in Australia is much more advanced than in other industrialised countries: Australia in the 1990s might turn out to be the California of the 1970s.

Not only has this book been written in the right place, but also at the right time. During the 1970s and 1980s most western babies were born in an electronic environment. Recently many studies compared groups of women giving birth with electronic foetal monitoring versus groups of women giving birth with a midwife listening to the baby's heart beats now and then. All these studies, published in the most authoritative medical journals, agreed that the only significant effect of the use of electronics during labour is to increase the rate of caesarean and forceps deliveries. There is no significant difference between the two groups when one compares the number of babies alive at birth and the number of babies healthy at birth. So, according to the most serious and orthodox medical literature, there is no reason for all babies to be born in an electronic environment. More generally speaking, the time has come to wonder about the effects of the environment on the process of birth, and the first contact between mother and baby. In other words, we are at the dawn of the post-electronic age.

To prepare for the post-electronic age we must first preserve the positive advances of this century in the field of childbirth. One of the main advances is the current technique of caesarean section. A modern caesarean section is a wonderful rescue operation. It should not become accepted as a way to be born. We have also to learn from our main mistakes. The electronic mirage is one of them; another was the assumption that a woman has to learn to give birth.

But, first of all, we have to go back to our deepest roots and remember that we are mammals. While studying for nearly 30 years the effect of the environment on the process of birth either in a hospital setting or at home, I became more and more convinced of the need for this awareness. We share with other mammals the same basic needs where birth is concerned. Most mammals tend to hide themselves, to isolate themselves to give birth and welcome their babies; their basic need is privacy. It is the same for humans. You can reach the same conclusions by reading carefully the stories of births collected by David. One of the highlights of the book is the birth of Daniel, the 'boy in a hurry'. All the conditions were met for an easy and fast birth. Sue was kneeling by her bed at night, probably in the dark, while her husband was asleep on the other side of the bed. Another highlight of the book (which has many highlights!) is the warning by Kristie, when writing about her 'exhaustion after childbirth': 'Limit your visitors to none or the absolute bare minimum, which may very well be easier said than done'.

Not only have we to remember that we are mammals but also that we are special mammals: we are aquatic apes. Compare humans with the other mammals and you will find dozens of obvious differences: we are naked; we have subcutaneous fat; we have salty tears; we have a large brain; we are orgasmic and we copulate face to face; we cannot be totally healthy without consuming some seafood; we have a diving reflex, etc. All these differences either mean adaptation to the sea or are a common point with the sea mammals. I learnt a lot about our aquatic nature by observing the strong attraction to water many labouring women have.

I hope that many readers throughout the world will improve their understanding of human nature by reading *Birth at Home*.

This book is one of the stones we need with which to lay the foundations of the post-electronic era.

Michel Odent

Life is short and the Art long; opportunity fleeting; evidence uncertain, experiment dangerous; experience deceptive and judgment difficult.

Hippocrates
Father of medicine, 400BC

Introduction

'There's no place like home,' said Steve, a recent home birth dad, about his experience. Indeed, the history of home birth goes back into antiquity, to the cave of our origins. We have been born in mansions, hovels, boats and gypsy vans — all places under the sun. The difference nowadays is the medical knowledge and technology which makes birth safer. Surely everyone has an equal right to the privilege of safe childbirth.

The trend to birth in hospital is relatively recent, really only in the last fifty to sixty years. Most mothers, of course, opt for this way, but a determined minority believe that birth is not an illness and can be safely conducted at home.

The national home birth rate hovers around one per cent and seems to be rising. It's worth noting that in the Byron Shire of northern New South Wales this figure is now around 15 per cent. With the Green movement reaching middle Australia, this shift is likely to continue into other places.

Recently an eminent researcher caused a stir in international obstetric circles. He predicted that 'home birth will soon be accepted as a fact of life'. This was reported in a magazine circulated to all G.P.s, the *Australian Dr Weekly*. Professor Mont Liggins, from the National Women's Hospital in Auckland, told the British Congress of Obstetricians and Gynaecologists in London that 'support services must be made available to make births outside hospital as safe as possible'.

To help demystify home birth mothers, fathers, even a couple of grandmothers present at births share their experiences and feelings in this book. Birth, being part of life's reality, sometimes means hardship and sadness. But most of the stories are joyful and there are some surprises too. The stories are written from the heart. They are personal accounts from a series of births starting as far back as 1979, happening mostly at home. Some hospital births are included.

When asked to contribute, some women expressed lack of confidence in their ability to write. But a spirit of caring for the mothers coming after them in labour provided a strong motive for the stories which follow. My experience as a birth doctor is here to show how I resolved my own doubts and uncertainties to come to understand the wonder of

INTRODUCTION

natural birth. The same questions and fears which assailed me, I still hear expressed: 'But what if something goes wrong at home?' So I hope the information in these stories is helpful.

The stories are edited from a professional viewpoint and so there are practical tips. In no way is this book a 'how-to' manual, though some of the recollections clearly point 'how not-to'.

Certain common birth procedures were found through experience to be completely unnecessary. Woman after woman said 'no episiotomy' (cutting the woman's vagina to let the baby out more quickly). Although this leaves a neater, easier cut to stitch than an accidental tear, it can cause long term painful scarring. Old episiotomies often 'unzip' at subsequent births. A spontaneous tear, if it occurs at all, seems to heal with a better result. The tissues are not cut 'across the grain', but give way across natural tissue layers. Just one example, to show that in the rapidly changing field of childbirth, we need to be open to the possibilities, not just locked into old prejudice. In such ways I discovered over time that the women know what they require.

Birth more than any other field in medicine requires a blending of art and science, and so methods need to be continually evaluated. The mode of some of these births may seem odd, even eccentric. but each one was backed up with medical safety: the presence of a doctor or qualified midwife carrying equipment as the ground rule.

The statistics behind these stories were looked at in retrospect and found comparable to other home birth statistics from Australia and overseas. The results of a recent survey in Western Australia are included for comparison.

The feelings behind the statistics are crystallised through the lens of John McCormick, the invisible witness to these events. His photographs provide a focus for the stories.

The writers were chosen at random, depending on who was around at the time. One mother, Elsbeth, agreed to write as she and I met crossing the street one day a few years after her birthing.

The water medium in labour figures largely in these stories. Its effectiveness in pain relief and relaxation during labour is so obvious that demand is increasing all the time. Some families go to great lengths to organise the water, as not every home has a bath built in. In some of these water labours, the mother is so comfortable she says 'why move?' and

INTRODUCTION

delivers her baby underwater. This element attracted international interest as a result of the work undertaken in the hospital of a French provincial market town. In June 1983, at Pithiviers, Dr Michel Odent and his team of midwives reported their one hundredth birth under water, with a perfect safety record (*Lancet*, December 1983).

Like Odent, I have found the working birth team to be a mainstay of good management. Midwives and trained supporters need to be involved right through from early pregnancy to form close bonds with the mother for the birth and that most important couple of weeks after the birth.

Home birth was a new experience for every member of this now established flexible team. Two of these supporters, Pam Sonia and Jude Holland, have been with the team for five years and their stories are woven through these tales of birth. There is no doubt about demand and interest in home birth; several doctors in this area have attended home births as a result of patient pressure. Some use this team for support.

Home birth work is rewarding and satisfying. Strong local support for the service gives encouragement to continue, but being on call is very draining. Labour can start at any time of day or night, anytime two weeks before or after the expected date. When it does start all the business of normal life has to be dropped, no matter how inconvenient. Burnout of childbirth personnel is common. Finding replacements is almost impossible, because very few midwives are trained or willing to work in the field.

Communication in this spread-out rural mountainous settlement is a challenge always. A ground rule before accepting a planned home birth is the installation of a working telephone in the home.

A survey in 1985 showed that home birth accounted for more than 20 per cent of the total in this shire. At the time this was forty times the national average. What makes the difference? Lifestyle is one thing. The area is a living laboratory of social change and a crystal ball into future trends. Also it seems that wherever an integrated home birth service is offered, such a service is well patronised.

'But what if something unexpectedly goes wrong?' This question is asked again and again, being one of the central concerns of any responsible person about birth at home. There are various ways to look at this. Things can go awry even in hospital. As far as home goes, essential safety means care and attention as well as proper planning by qualified and

INTRODUCTION

experienced people, who carry the right equipment to the place of birth, which is always visited beforehand. This is called 'taking the hospital to the home'.

If transfer to hospital for essential treatment is required it is arranged by telephone. Difficulties with such a transfer can occur if some ultra-conservative birth professional in the hospital is trying to prove a point. I have seen labouring women deliberately punished. It seems that such occurrences are becoming less common with better understanding that childbirth is not an illness. Having a baby is different to the removal of the appendix and hospitals are becoming more aware of people's right to choose.

Changing attitudes to birth are being pioneered by the women and men who have the courage to stand up for the right to conduct their own family affairs. It is only by continuing to listen to them that we can continue to support the process of change for the better. In particular, more and more we are learning something about the post natal period — that forgotten time when problems which can get out of hand may be prevented by timely measures.

But let's start at the beginning…

Looking Back
A Doctor's Personal Journey

Everyone contributing to this book has written a personal story. This is mine and aims to recall the unexpected way I became involved in natural childbirth.

That first encounter with childbirth stands out as a high point for the medical student of the late 60s. After all the dry lectures and tutorials, it was the first real taste at being a doctor.

On with the gown and gloves to actually touch a patient, to do something — getting a baby out. My first instructor was a midwife rather than a doctor. Years of births later I have become aware of the vital importance of good midwifery to the mother's and baby's welfare. The midwife, a highly qualified person, is labour's guide. A word in the right place from her can save the day. Sometimes, with the right help, a mother can be spared the first step in that all-too-familiar cascade of intervention, and progress to a natural birth.

Anyway, to return, this very senior and experienced midwife emanated confidence which was contagious; and made me, the anxious student, feel okay at my first birth.

'Get the chin,' she said, and showed me a technique which involved grinding my knuckles into the woman's backside to stop the baby's head from slipping back between contractions.

I was determined not to lose the chin, lest the baby slip up away from my grasp altogether. I might still be there if I hadn't got the chin. Later on I realised this was my first lesson in unnecessary intervention. There was not much consideration taught for the feelings of the woman behind the baby. But this particular midwife also taught me a good lesson in humility. 'The most important thing,' she said, 'is cleaning up afterwards. Here's the mop.'

Of all my student days, the most remarkable part was a three month elective term spent in a remote New Guinea mission on Bougainville Island. The usual doctor went on leave as soon as I arrived.

As they couldn't get a suitably qualified replacement doctor they had to settle for me. I soon found out how little I knew about medicine. I didn't see any birth because it was all conducted in the villages by local native midwives. The people were afraid of the hospital.

So I saw one case only, a complication. A woman with puerperal (afterbirth) fever arrived from the village in quite a bad way. 'If only,' we said, 'they had their babies here in the mission hospital, there wouldn't be these complications.' In retrospect, I realised I was behaving as a hospital doctor criticising home birth, because the only aspect I saw was a complication.

Looking right back, I was one of five children, and grew up in the 50s under the influence of a strong father, an illustrious doctor. My father, a pioneer in the field of neurosurgery, was always busy and often away. Medical visitors from Australia and abroad frequently came to the home and we children became used to different faces and accents at an early age. But in the midst of this situation was the freedom to explore. We had horses, dogs and local bush to enjoy, with creeks, waterholes and wildlife. The constant presence of our loving mother was as natural as the sun rising each morning. I suppose, looking back, we were a privileged lot.

Now, attending birth at home is part of my everyday working life. It wasn't always like that. So it's interesting to reflect on changes that led to a doctor arising from such an established medical background eventually becoming involved in the controversial area of home birth in the country town of Mullumbimby, a place with a difference which will become apparent.

In 1970 I finished my student days and was allocated Newcastle for internship. Some of my other new doctor friends with better exam results were sent to teaching hospitals in the city. This seemed to be a setback but later I realised how fortunate I was, as the opportunities for learning practical skills were far greater in country centres. It became apparent from friends who stayed that much of the direction in establishment centres was geared towards jockeying for position and status. So this start suited me well, as I wished later to travel abroad for further experience and training, the eventual aim to settle somewhere as a country G.P. This is what happened, but country practice turned out rather differently than I envisaged at the time.

That year of internship incidentally can be a shock for the fledgling doctor, suddenly plunged into unaccustomed responsibility and decision-making, which affects the welfare of patients, including life and death decisions way beyond his competence or experience.

I recall the frustrations of dealing with some common conditions which didn't seem to be acknowledged in textbooks. Many lower back pain patients, for example, went away unrelieved by standard investigations and treatment. I heard references to the quaint oriental practice of acupuncture. Also I heard of patients being miraculously and instantly cured by manipulation. But discussion of such practices in the 60s was brushed aside. Mostly not discussed at all.

It seemed to me that a most important role for the doctor was to find the methods which most helped the patient. I didn't know at the time about wholistic healing. In fact the term hadn't even been invented. My only tools were still the orthodox methods, handed down. There was never a serious question that there might be other ways.

But obstetrics was the most exciting field, because of the

dynamic nature of the birth process. The challenge of surgical obstetrics was even more absorbing. I recall the first occasion, watching the great master apply obstetrical forceps with aplomb to the baby's head. Quite awe-inspiring to one who had never seen such a thing done.

Although the way he then put one foot on the end of the bed and tugged and tugged until the baby emerged at first filled me with some anticipation that one day the baby's head might just emerge not attached to its poor little body. I was reassured though, that the baby would not be harmed by this procedure, so felt compelled to learn this technique and made myself available for every opportunity.

Later on, a more sensitive obstetrician taught me how to use traction on the forceps only while the woman's uterus was contracting, thus pulling, to assist her pushing. This approach seemed to make better sense, as forceps could be used more gently, but used nevertheless.

Now my perceptions have changed so much that avoiding the use of forceps on the unborn baby is a definite aim of management.

In those earlier days after I had attended quite a few births the normal delivery was not so interesting. There was nothing much to do. Hard to justify being there. To me at the time, the learning experience gained from involvement with a complicated delivery was what I was seeking to help me in the future when I would be on my own. But looking for trouble made it occur more frequently, I'm sure.

The intern year finished and I was developing confidence in my basic skills. My dad tried to encourage me back into the teaching hospitals, but I had been at school long enough and felt like seeing the world. I realised that by going away I would sacrifice my chances of real career success as a specialist. But that didn't matter, because I had decided to be a country doctor anyway. Maybe I felt the need to get away. My sister Kathy tossed me a remark along these lines: 'For the little acorn to grow, far from the mighty chestnut must it go.'

The next episode didn't do much for my medical education but got me to England and a supply of anecdotes: a job as ship's doctor on an old cargo ship. The trip, for which I was paid a shilling, took five weeks.

My inspection of the ship's pharmacy filled me with anxiety and misgivings as I, a modern doctor, did not recognise any of the antique medicines on board. So, in a spirit of responsibility I went ashore before sailing and ordered some medicines I was more familiar with and booked them up to the line. At Panama I was summoned before the captain who had been informed of my shopping spree. He was furious and boomed at me in a Scottish accent: 'Have yer gooot yer cheque boook with yer Doctor?' I need not have worried because the sailors seemed to know what they wanted anyway.

On board there were several large glass jars equipped with little taps. One of these was labelled 'Black Draught'. It was not listed in any book, but was issued on request to seamen who carried their own glasses into the clinic. Not wishing to appear ignorant, it took a couple of weeks on board to discover its true nature. This mixture contained bromide, used for the purpose of helping crewmen relax their sexual desires at sea.

Prior to my row with the captain, I had developed a daily routine of going to the bridge to learn some navigation. The second mate kindly taught me how to use the sextant to perform sun sights. One day he was taking a noon sight, sextant in one hand, cigarette in the other. The 'old man' strictly forbade smoking on the bridge. 'He's coming,' urgently whispered the lookout and the panicked mate threw his sextant overboard. As the captain appeared a moment later he shouted, 'What are ye doing smoking on my bridge?'

I was glad to leave the ship of fools in England where I walked into a job in Anaesthetics and Intensive Care, otherwise known as 'expensive scare'. Here I met the experienced and canny Dr Middleton Price who taught me how to relax in urgent situations.

'Always walk to an emergency,' he advised. 'Never run'. The unflustered doctor is more use and inspires confidence in calmness. I never forgot that and it became important to the way I try to practise in everyday life.

After travelling and working abroad I still wanted to be a country doctor, so it was back to Newcastle and a job offer at the Western Suburbs Maternity Hospital which gave me a chance to sit for the Diploma in Obstetrics in the early 70s. I already had a fair grounding but needed a lot more practice and got plenty of it there.

In many ways looking back, the intensive training was at odds with the practice I now engage in and aspire to.

In those days there was never any objection or questioning by the mother. For instance, forceps delivery was the order of the day for dealing with any delay and all I had to remember were the obstetric rules:

- the cervix is fully dilated;
- the bladder is empty;
- the membranes must be ruptured;
- the head is engaged;
- the position must be ascertained;
- a wide episiotomy must be performed.

So much of what we were doing was all about intervention. Starting with catheterisation of the bladder and of course the necessary anaesthetic. Needless to say the whole performance was quite painful, but to me at the time, that's just the way things were done.

Two other common customs are worth mentioning:
'Monitoring' is the practice of attaching a machine to the mother and baby to record accurately each contraction and heartbeat. A new art, it was becoming very popular and I can remember the first monitor at my hospital, which created a lot of interest, and became regarded as almost indispensable for a truly safe labour. It gave the doctor a good feeling of total control over every aspect of the

mother and baby and I was very interested in this development. It was often difficult for the mother to be comfortable all wired up, but everybody was very reassured by being able to watch the tracings on the screen. Any irregularity could be attended to early with appropriate action. The caesarian and forceps rate climbed alarmingly, but the babies were born in good condition.

Surprisingly, more recent evaluation of monitoring has shown that the practice does not improve infant welfare. A report by the respected National Health and Medical Research Council states that '...There is no evidence that routine foetal monitoring has a positive effect on the outcome of pregnancy. Electronic foetal monitoring should be carried out only in carefully selected cases related to high perinatal mortality rates and where labour is induced. Research should investigate the selection of women who might benefit from foetal monitoring. Meanwhile, national health services should abstain from purchasing new equipment. It is recommended that the foetal heart be monitored through auscultation [listening through a stethoscope] during the first stage of labour, and more frequently during expulsion...'

Another common practice to consider is that of induction, which has in recent years received a lot of adverse publicity. The rationale for inducing (artificially starting labour) is if rescue of the baby from the mother's womb seems necessary. The real reason sometimes has to do with the convenience of the staff or even the mother.

I remember the induction days well. Sometimes it worked without any problem, but all too often the mother seemed unripe and the induction didn't work. Caesarian section follows failed induction.

The epidural nerve block, which causes numbing below the waist, was becoming commonly used and seemed to be the really only completely painfree method of performing procedures, whilst allowing the woman to stay awake. The magic of the epidural became apparent in its usefulness to actually avoid forcep procedures. A real windfall this, because for some reason, after the epidural was administered, if a little time was allowed to elapse, the labour would very often proceed by itself to completion. Even the obstinate cervix would dilate and avoid the need for some caesarians as well as forceps.

How can this procedure which blocks sensation from the woman's pelvis have its own positive effect on labour? It's hard to explain, but I see it this way. Tension and raw fear coming from the woman's mind can inhibit labour. If this negative force is overcome (by the anaesthetic nerve block), the natural process can go forward. Seen in perspective, there is a lesson to be learned from this experiment. If fear can truly interfere with labour, then, how much more can childbirth without fear be truly enhanced rather than impeded by the natural process?

It was only later I began to realise the desirability of avoiding interference. For example, even though the force involved in a good forceps delivery may not leave any visible marks on the baby, beyond some bruising on the temples, who knows how the procedure may affect the baby's brain? After all, forceps delivery is a critical and exacting job. Any miscalculation of the baby's position can mean the blades go over his or her poor little face with unsightly results. These thoughts led me to what I now simply believe, namely, that our job as doctors or midwives is to not interfere unless absolutely necessary.

Years later the poem on the next page came into my hands and it reminded me of that chapter of my life, when I was very much part of the system that did not recognise the suffering. It was written by a woman called Caroline Denigan, but to me it stands as the poem of the unknown mother, whose lament needs to be listened to, now.

During my post-graduate training in the early 70s, I met a great doctor, Steele Fitchett, who has now retired from obstetrics and is involved in the care of the dying. His throwaway comment etched itself into my brain and would not go away: 'Childbirth,' he said, 'is

Imogene's Birth

How can I welcome you child?
In this atmosphere where I feel unwelcome
In a strange bed
Surrounded by unfamiliar, hostile faces
The face I know and love shoved aside
The other family faces sit and wait outside
Not allowed to witness your arrival
I feel cut off — dismembered.

Harsh white walls and overhead lights, glaring, blazing at us.
Am I the enemy — the dirt — the problem to be solved — dissolved?
Cold hard stainless steel robs me of my warmth.
Little wonder I want the pain to cease, my labour to stop,
you to remain safe within.

Bound to this table we can't escape the brutal prodding;
The fierce gaze of those who would deliver you from me.
They bear down on me hoping to force me to expel you.

I become tense when threatened with the knife,
Ensuring it will be wielded upon me;
Why can't they help me relax instead of paralysing me with fear?
Massage and soothe tense muscles
Instead of cutting through my resistance
At last you show yourself — wanting the ordeal to be over,
Hoping they will then leave us alone.
But the masked bandits wait to take you from me,
Deserted, humiliated, wounded to the heart,
How can I welcome you child?

Caroline Denigan

a family affair.'

At some of his births, I even saw some husbands present, at the time practically unheard of. None of them fainted or went bananas. Mostly they were quite over-awed and very well behaved and grateful to be there. Fitchett, I noticed, even had some of his women sitting propped up, with pillows behind for labour. I had never seen a doctor pay attention to 'positioning' as a factor in easing birth trauma.

Sometime after I asked the very experienced Dr Ferguson, an old style G.P., and a master of the dry understatement, if anyone ever had their babies at home? 'They used to,' he said, 'occasionally I still am asked and carry a pair of forceps in the bottom of my bag, which I never have to use anyway.'

It didn't hit me then, but he was telling me something about home birth, which meant something about less intervention. In general home birth was not a subject much discussed, being somewhat taboo — anyway there was never a hospital bed shortage and so no need. The only reference was to the 'Flying Squad', a British phenomenon of which we had no equivalent in Australia (in Britain, of course, having babies at home has been part of established medical practice for years)

After finishing the diploma, came the offer of a job in Lismore, a regional city, which was to soon lead me to Mullumbimby. The turning point came in Intensive Care one weekend. A child arrived covered in mud, apparently lifeless after an accident in a dam. The six year old, while playing with his friend on their place in the hills behind Mullumbimby, had slipped into the muddy water and disappeared. His little friend ran to the house and found the dad, Bill, who ran down and after some time discovered his son's inert body half buried in mud.

How long was he under? At least twenty minutes it was later calculated. A lightning dash to Mullumbimby (half an hour) found no doctor available, and so a further drive to Lismore (another three-quarters of an hour) had the exhausted party arriving muddy, wet and half dressed at the doors of Lismore hospital. We instigated emergency procedures and by some miracle Adam's vital functions were restored.

No doubt the continuing resuscitation efforts by his father in the back of his speeding station wagon helped to save the day. Still, there was no sign of consciousness for a couple of days and the outlook was gloomy. Having to tell the parents was very difficult.

But by the end of the second day, there were unmistakable signs of recovery and by the third day Adam was trying to pull the tube out of his throat. He made a complete recovery and I have seen him from time to time over the years, completely intelligent and functional. Adam now has a younger sister which I helped his mother deliver years later in Mullumbimby hospital.

Apart from the wonderment of this child's survival, there was a significant meeting. At his bedside I met Sylvia, who asked me to deliver her baby in Mullumbimby — the first of several hundred deliveries in the district. Sylvia's determination to have her baby naturally was to completely alter my approach to childbirth.

BYRON SHIRE

A visit to this charming area of beautiful clean surf beaches and rainforest hinterland had me convinced to go there to work and set up a practice. At that time Mullumbimby was a typical sleepy Australian country town, except for the recent influx of 'hippies', who were all flat to the boards buying up 'rubbish country' so called by local farmers many of whom were selling up due to the demise of the dairy industry.

I suppose I should have guessed that the attitude to childbirth might be different to the norm when I looked around the district. As I was taken around to meet the new settlers the profusion and variety of dwellings hidden in the bush of the hills amazed me. A round house, a hexagonal dome covered all over with quaint shingles, a house built with a tree growing through the roof, just to

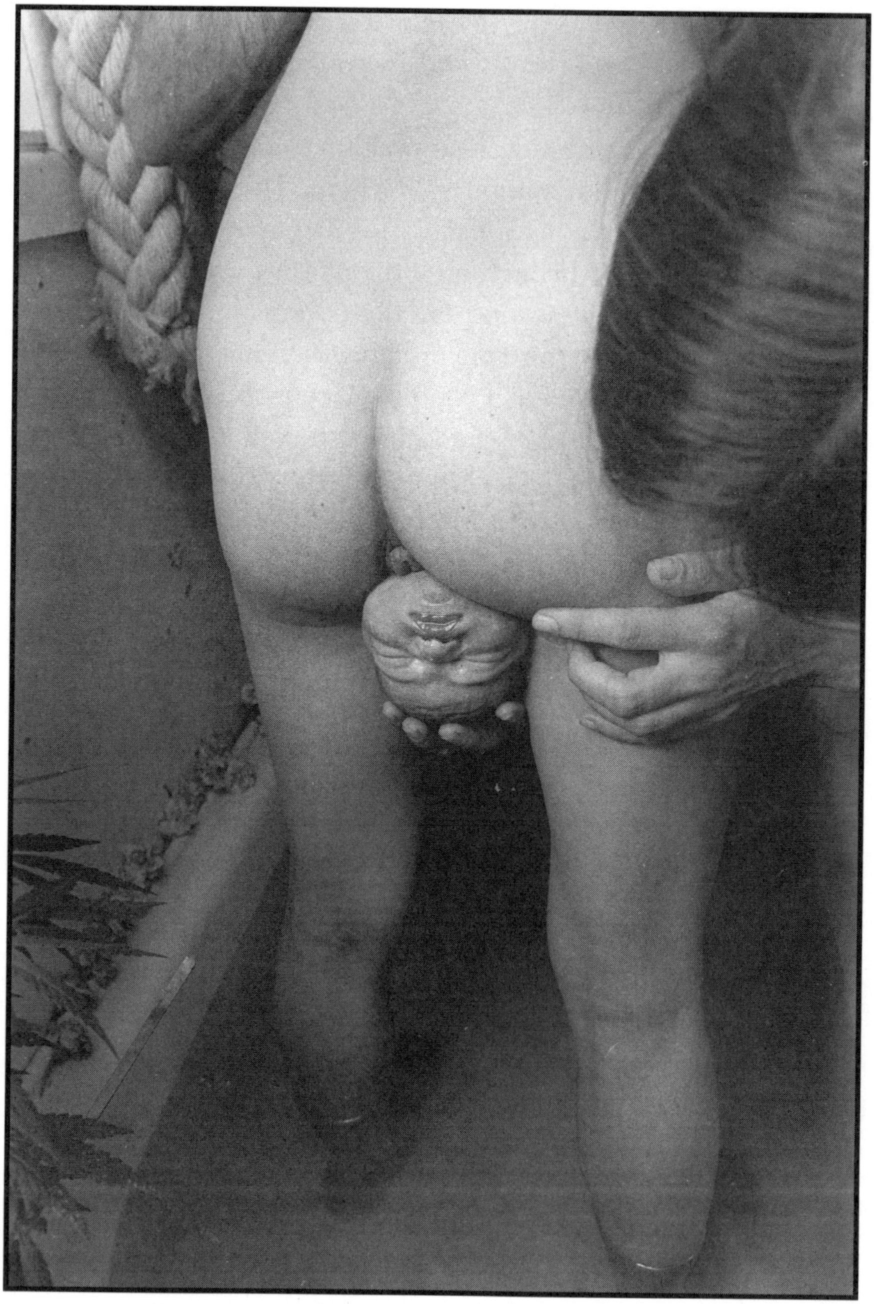

BIRTH AT HOME

BIRTH AT HOME

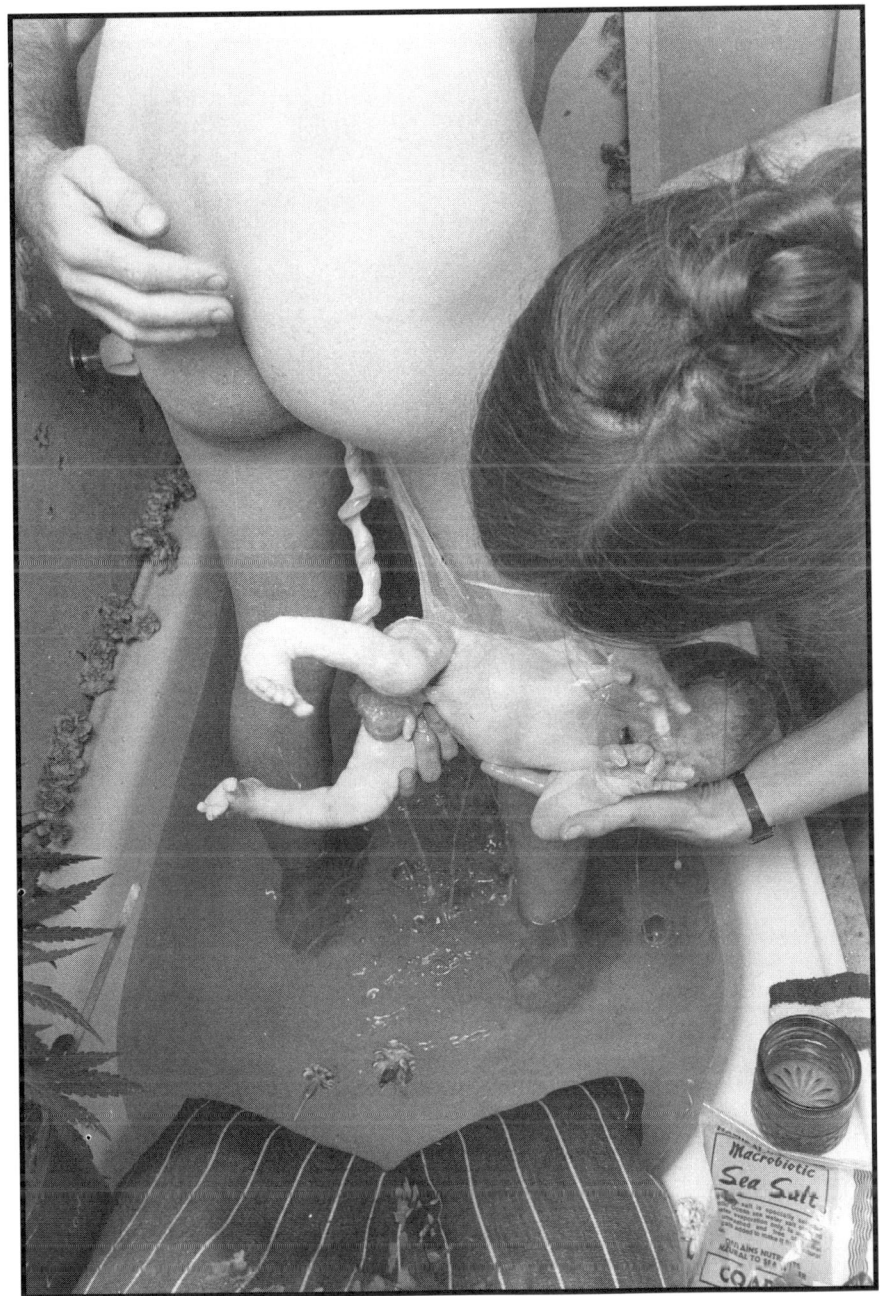

BIRTH AT HOME

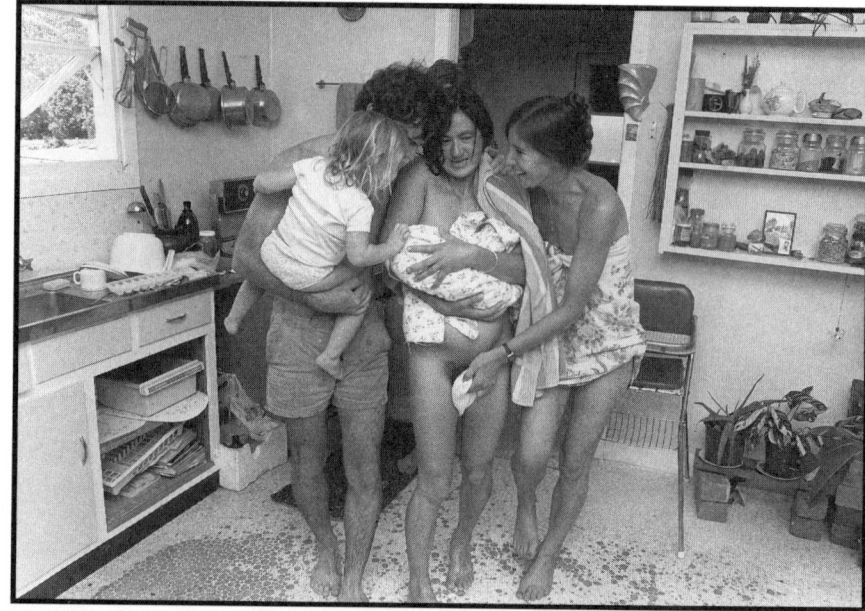

The joy and pure energy that fills the room or birth space the moment the new little one arrives never ceases to fill me with miraculous wonder.

JUDE, MIDWIFE

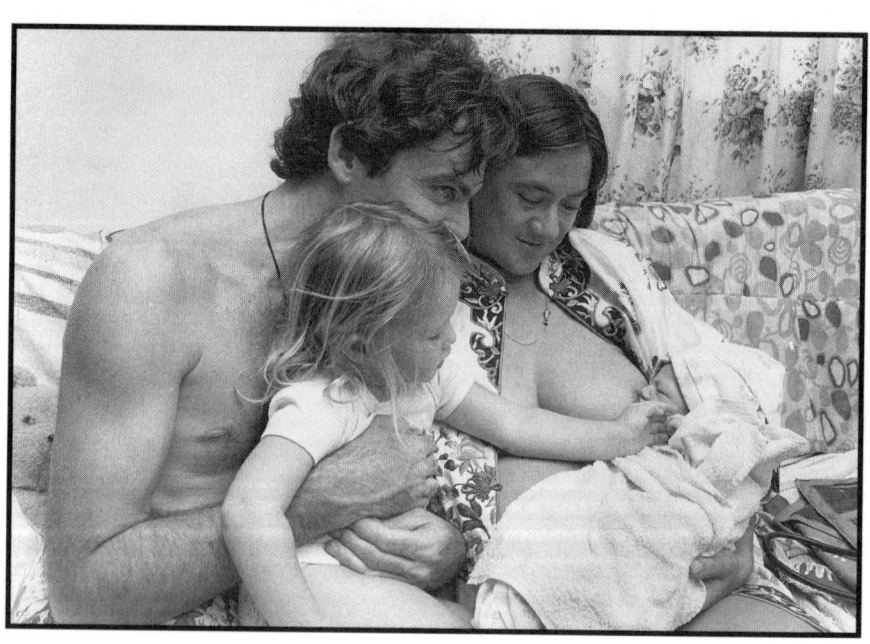

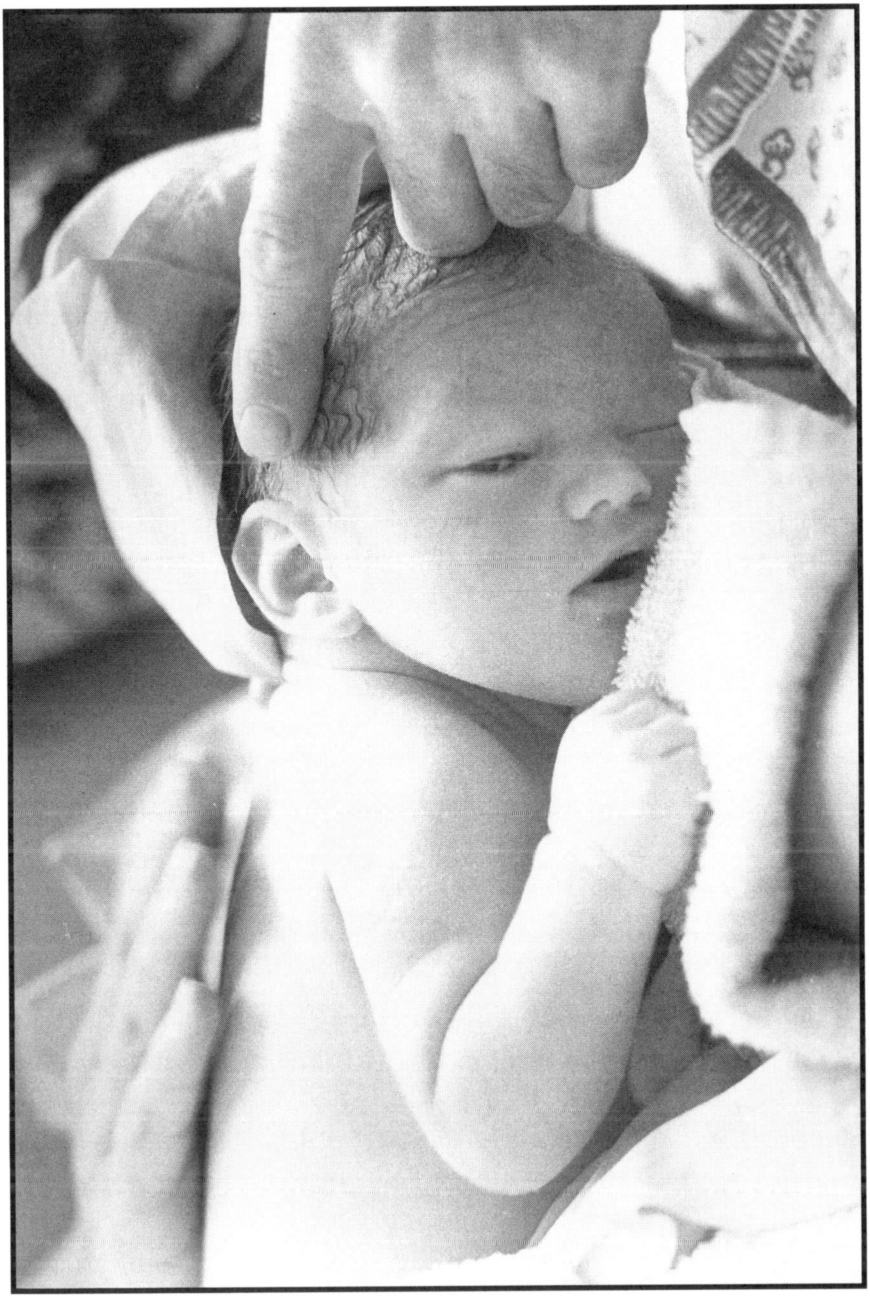

BIRTH AT HOME

Home birth is great theatre. It has all the elements of high drama—romance, a hero, the heroine, courage, fortitude and devotion, a strong supporting cast and a dedicated stage director.

The real hero, finally revealed in the last act, is the baby. Graciously sharing the spotlight at the curtain call this child prodigy appears with the mother on one hand and the father on the other. the stage managers, the doctor and midwife take a bow from the wings while parents, grandparents, relatives and assorted friends deliver a standing ovation. The stage managers retire with a grand glow of satisfaction to observe and, when necessary, to assist in the many sequels that are bound to follow.

FRANK, GRANDFATHER

mention a few.

My new rooms were in an old office which had not been occupied for ten years. It was full of old rubbish and spiderwebs. The front window was broken and the roof leaked, but the walls were lined with cedar panels taken from the wreck of the Byron-Sydney ferry — the *Wollongbar* — a beautiful ship which grounded before she could get up steam by a storm years before in Byron Bay. A retired (young) nurse, Marie, appeared from her shingle dome in the hills to become my first loyal secretary.

The growing population of new settlers, hippies, hill tribes and alternatives formed an instant backbone to my practice and I was busy immediately. But I was in for some shocks.

'No, I don't want drugs and chemicals' and 'I don't want to be cut open either'. At first I got annoyed but soon came to see that these people wanted another way, and that's why they were here.

I had to learn something new, and I kept learning from these people. It was one of them who told me about Frederick Leboyer and showed me his recent book, *Birth Without Violence*. This book and its influence swept the Western world, including our district and the demand for non-violent childbirth was starting to be heard. Leboyer writes: 'But is birth really so important? people may ask. It doesn't last long, in comparison with what precedes and follows, it's just a nasty moment to be got through. That, I think, is somewhat glib. After all, there is another "nasty moment" which, though possibly equally brief, nonetheless casts a long shadow: that of death. Birth may be a matter of a moment. But it is a unique one. To be born means to begin to breathe, to embark on that perpetual motion which will be with us until we die. Our breathing is a fragile vessel that carries us from birth to death. Everyone breathes...'

Thoughts like this provided a good reason to pursue the ideal of conscious birth; to give the newborn an opportunity for a good start in life. Seeing the baby as a sensitive, aware individual with feelings, rights and prospects, made me aware of the terrible struggle involved not only for the mother, who could complain, but the unborn baby, who could not.

By trying to see through the eyes of the newborn, Dr Leboyer pointed out that to arrive with rough handling, facing a bright focused light, after forty weeks in watery darkness is a cruel shock. To be immediately separated from the heart sound and feel of the mother must be very anxiety provoking and indeed disorienting.

This concept reinforced for me the notion of using obstetric forceps as something to be avoided if at all possible. 'We never touch the head', says Leboyer. From here, for me there was no turning back, and bit by bit, under the guidance of my watchful patients, I learned to simplify, simplify. All the time learning how to do away with unnecessary procedures.

But of course while learning from the patients was one thing, I came to understand that such changes inevitably meant crossing swords with officialdom.

The first battle of many with the local health services concerned the issue of father in the labour room. 'But most of them are not even married,' complained the matron. 'We can't have that, they can look through the glass in the door if they must, but they can't come in. We have to think of sterility.'

As I turned to walk away, defeated, she said: 'Only husbands and then only if they sign an agreement.' What luck, Sylvia and Graham were actually married. Tough on the outside, this old matron had her heart in the right place, and Sylvia had her baby — my first delivery at Mullumbimby — with Graham joyfully at her side in the hospital.

Many prospective parents asked for home birth, but at this stage I did not believe that such a practice could be safe and always said, 'No, we can do natural birth just as well in hospital.'

An old experienced local G.P., Dr Guy Ethell, taught me many skills, showing me that medical learning did not finish, but was really beginning out in practice. He taught me to be confident and do things for myself, rather than referring everything to specialists. Given what lay ahead, this confidence was to prove invaluable.

It was on house calls to the hills that I came to know the district. Finding a house could be quite a riddle as there are no house numbers and few street names. Many settlers deliberately built their houses in hidden seclusion.

My pregnant patients became a special interest and I learned to listen to their demands, outrageous as they often seemed at the time. Still, I did listen and over a period of time learned that a more harmonious labour resulted when I:

- switched off the bright lights;
- reduced my own and other people's noise level;
- made husbands and children welcome;
- encouraged a support person, usually a female friend;
- reduced dress formality, and;
- used less drugs.

Small things, but altogether they added up to a very different kind of experience.

It seemed that whenever I was around pregnant women, there was always a lot of talk about the feelings of the baby. There was even talk about the mother squatting to deliver. That I could handle. But home birth was still a big 'No No'. After all it was obviously not safe, or so I still thought. As for water birth, well, not even the hippies talked about that in the mid-70s.

I didn't realise it at the time, but I was lucky enough to be involved in the forefront of the birth revolution, a movement which was gathering steam in the whole Western world as part of the cultural change reflected in the moods of music, lifestyle and a desire to return to nature.

After a year in Mullumbimby, I was faced with a landmark dilemma. One of my patients was having her first child. The baby was due, and still the head had not engaged. According to normal practice, I arranged a pelvimetry examination. This is an X-ray to determine whether the baby's head would fit through the mother's pelvis. I was very disappointed when the report came back that it could not — the mother's pelvis was too small. So I advised her that she would need a caesarian.

She burst into tears and asked me if there was any other way. I remembered some advice that Dr Fitchett had once given me: 'Nearly everybody is entitled to a chance in labour. What is there to lose?' So I told her we could start labour but not to be too disappointed if it didn't work out.

When labour started a few days later this woman wouldn't stay on the bed and walked around the labour room. She squatted down on the floor during contractions. Much to my surprise, the baby's head engaged and she started dilating her cervix. After a straightforward labour she delivered a beautiful baby in good condition; squatting on the bed.

Measuring the bony pelvis with an X-ray is a very static and arbitrary judgment and does not seem to take into account the very real benefits of freeing the woman from lying on her back on the operating table. I learned in the most obvious way that a woman's position can be greatly significant in helping her deliver with ease. This experience affirmed for me the woman's right to a realistic trial of labour.

Testing the edges of the 'rules' creates a lot of anxiety, but winning without intervention under those conditions is a great victory for the mother and baby, as well as the doctor and midwife!

Once again it was a patient who handed me something obvious and important. Another thing I was coming to understand at this time was the importance of allowing enough time for the natural processes to evolve. Allowing this time while keeping a close unobtrusive eye on the mother and baby requires a very cautious approach and it was from experience that I began to privately extend the laid down times for different stages of labour. 'Half an hour for a multi, and one hour for a primip in second stage' had been washed into my brain during training. To my great satisfaction I was now finding that these times could be extended without damage. I came to a conclusion that labour which is progressing and rhythmical is safe, provided that the baby's heartbeat is regular. This is easily checked at intervals with the portable doppler foetal stethoscope, as recommended by the National Health and Medical Research Council. Foetal distress under these conditions is extremely rare.

HOME CARE MEDICINE

In the early 80s, while spending some time working in Cairns in North Queensland, I had my first contact with community support groups, in particular a home birth support group and the cancer support group. I became more involved in looking after people at home in birth, death and illness with the very able support of the Blue Nursing Association of Queensland. We even managed intravenous drips and blood transfusions within the home.

With this support I learned the art of 'taking the hospital to the home'. We didn't do major operations at home like they did in the early 1900s, as my father recalls in his book *A Surgeon's Story*. He remembers accompanying his chief, Sir Alexander McCormick, into the homes of the very rich in Sydney in two Rolls Royces all loaded down with surgical equipment, including an operating table!

Home in those days was considered safer, even for major operations, because there was less incidence of post-operative wound infection than in the hospital. Isn't it interesting they knew way back then that recovery was faster in the patient's own home, in the company of familiar people, food and surroundings. Naturally the expenses were very high, as constant nursing and home visits by the doctor were required.

Unfortunately, the cost aspect of home care is still a problem today. People who choose home birth have to expect to pay more for all the aftercare required. There's no getting round the need, for example, for extra domestic help.

It's a pity the government doesn't acknowledge the great opportunity for savings that home birth and home care generally provides by reducing the need for expensive hospital care. Every home birth saves the tax payer thousands of dollars. A policy which offers extra health service and support devoted to domestic back-up and home nursing would mean not only a real saving to the health system but release hospital beds for cases that really need them.

Soon after engaging in home birth, I came to realise there was a lot of opposition within the profession to this practice, which caused me a good deal of distress and involved some tension with colleagues.

I asked my father his opinion on home birth and he told me, 'I can't see what's wrong with it. I was born at home. My father, your grandfather, Dr Joseph Miller used to attend home births in Brunswick, Victoria where he practised. He apparently used to go out on calls with a couple of old biddies who helped him.' That was nearly a hundred years ago. I also asked my mother her opinion. 'There was too much fuss about the childbirth process when I was having all of you,' she said.

PITHIVIERS

In the early 80s, I visited the clinic of Dr Michel Odent, a French doctor who practised natural childbirth and underwater birth in the town of Pithiviers, outside Paris. Odent worked freely in the obstetric wing of a normal provincial French hospital, a remarkable achievement and really a credit to the French health authorities that they allowed it to happen.

Dr Odent is a very wise and relaxed man who told me that as doctors 'Our job is to *not* interfere'. He expressed the idea that if a woman can return to her instinctive self in labour, then anxiety or fear is less likely to inhibit labour. A natural flow of hormones changes the consciousness and the woman feels, as he put it, 'as though she is on another planet'.

Odent indicated that women can find this state of mind very easily by climbing into a warm bath. Once in, as he pointed out to me, the woman often wants to stay there, saying 'why move?' and has her baby under the water.

So this was the next item — water birth — and those inevitable questions: 1) what about the baby? 2) how does it breathe? 3) what about infection? 4) can't the baby drown?

If the baby has been growing under water for forty weeks, it is not an unfamiliar environment and so it will not attempt to breathe air. The lungs are folded and can only be expanded by air. The placenta is still supplying oxygen and nutrients and the heart rate can be simply tested by feeling the cord. In any case, the baby usually comes quickly to the surface. You sometimes see babies frog swimming up to their mother's tummy.

Infection? Dr Odent explained that there is not time for organisms to grow and of course the water is clean to start with.

And 'why water anyway?' as I'm so frequently asked. Well that's so simple, really. After all, how does it feel after a long, world weary day to climb into a deep warm bath, to ease away all those aches and worries, to allow the mind to relax?

And some other considerations:

Human beings have an affinity to water and are attracted to pools, waterfalls, the ocean, and rivers. Any path you find meandering through the bush will nearly always end up at the water.

The first forty weeks of all our lives have been spent in the water of the womb.

Without water there can be no life on earth.

Eighty per cent of our body weight is water.

Swimming pools are commonly used for stroke and accident rehabilitation in hospitals — paralysed people can often swim, when walking is not possible.

The encounter with Odent was reassuring, confirming as it did my own experiences in Mullumbimby where there was a big and growing demand from women wanting to have their babies at home and many in fact opting for water birth.

The demand for home birth in the Mullumbimby region is very high. By 1985, 25 per cent of births in the Byron Shire were at home, compared with the national figure of less than 1 per cent.

Labour in water is a choice for many of the women whose stories appear here. The demand for this medium is becoming very popular. Because of the number of home births in our area, I was approached in 1987 by Dr Owen Spencer, a far-sighted administrative doctor of the regional health department, who foreshadowed a major review into birth practices in New South Wales. He asked me to prepare a report and attend conferences on changes in birth policies in New South Wales. This turned out to be really interesting because it showed me how many people were thinking along similar lines.

An obvious shift in community attitudes over the last few years is continuing. But the absorption of new values is so gradual that some of the things now taken for granted have been the scene of argument and confrontation between birth professionals and birthing families.

Many pregnant women that I see carry tales of horror from previous childbirth experiences — too many such stories indicate that there is still something seriously wrong with the standard system of childbirth delivery services.

That unnecessary cruelty and trauma to mother and babies is allowed to continue in a civilised society is hard to understand. The depth of the problem was expressed by Dr Odent who said, 'Obstetrics cannot be reformed. It must be replaced.' The good news is that changes are already being experienced. Among the changes:
- the father at the birth is now universally accepted;
- unnecessary obstetrical interference is seen as undesirable;
- routine use of drugs, e.g. vitamin K for the newborn, narcotics or nitrous oxide gas for the labouring mother, is questioned;
- the de-medicalisation of birth forms, pubic shaving, bright

lights, operating theatre costume for staff and family, is now considered old-fashioned;
- the concept of birth centres in hospitals has official acceptance and
- adoption of natural and active birth methods is seen as humane and sensible by increasing numbers of people.

Lots of mothers and their families see childbirth as a positive or a spiritual experience. The benefits to the baby of a non-violent and peaceful first step into this world should lead to the development of less violence in individuals and ultimately to the whole society. Otherwise why bother?

Knoweldg of birth is evolving fast. It's up to the health professions to keep up with the wishes of women, namely gentle birthing practices, allowing more time and less intervention.

As for me, looking back on how childbirth was and how it seems to me now, the differences are vast. Speeding to the hospital to catch a baby is a strange kind of custom. The quick and easy delivery hardly needs a doctor, whose services are more valuable to the baby who can't come out in such a hurry. A more relaxed and fruitful post-natal period is more likely to follow a smooth, unhurried and fulfilling birth. Post-natal depression under these conditions is quite uncommon.

MY CHILDREN — THE NOT THE HOME BIRTH STORY!

It will seem ironic that the children of a home birth practitioner should be born in hospital. But that was my wife's, Nean, choice, a choice which was mostly imposed by the fact that home birth practitioners were hard to find. I certainly didn't want to be the doctor either way.

Nean was lucky enough to have her babies in hospitals where there was a lot of supportive care and no interference. I enjoyed the luxury of not having the responsibility of the clinical side —

free to enjoy being a father.

NEAN'S STORY

David asked me to write about the birth of our children for possible inclusion in his home birth book. 'But,' I said, 'the kids were born in hospital!' David explained that he had asked many mothers to write their story and he felt it would be nice to include the births of his own children in his book. This made sense to me, so...

It may surprise you to learn that both my babies were born in hospitals. There were a number of reasons influencing the decision. David was only just coming round to the idea of home birth when our first child was due. I preferred him to be involved as the 'father' rather than the doctor. As no other doctors in the area were doing home birth, I decided it would be a hospital birth. David was a little disappointed that he wasn't going to deliver the child, but he finally understood my feelings on the necessity of his role of 'father/husband/supporter'.

Going back to the beginning — being pregnant was an absolute thrill to me. I read everything I could on the subject and prepared my body and mind for the big day. In the early stages of pregnancy I was diagnosed from a pap smear as having invasive cells (in other words, the early stages of cervical cancer). This frightened me indeed.

The doctor I was seeing advised me strongly to have the cancer removed there and then. I enquired if this would affect my pregnancy and he said there was a strong likelihood of the baby aborting itself. I decided not to have the operation as I was aware that the condition would not affect the unborn baby, and above all else I had no desire to lose my baby. I was well and truly ready for motherhood.

On a subsequent visit I was told my iron level was deficient and that I should take an iron supplement. I decided to eat lots of meals with fresh parsley and plenty of pumpkin. My iron reading was satisfactory after the next blood test.

My pregnancy progressed pleasantly and effortlessly. Two weeks before the due date, I awoke very early with the slightest trickle of amniotic fluid, followed by a very mild contraction — I thought 'here goes'. I had arranged for my Mother and Gayle, an extremely close friend, to be with me, as David was away.

A couple of hours passed by during which time my fluid kept trickling slowly and the contractions were building up at an even pace. We decided it was time to head for hospital.

On arrival, I was examined by a midwife who estimated that I had quite a way to go yet — I knew different. It only took another three hours. The doctor I had been seeing throughout my pregnancy was out of town on holidays. I was to have the doctor on call. This turned out fine — he was extremely helpful and in no way interfering. He knew I wanted to manage the birth myself.

The contractions continued to build up gradually. Before long I was experiencing heavy back pain. Mum and Gayle took turns to rub it, in the hope of relieving it. The moment they would stop rubbing, the pain would become almost unbearable. The poor things, I worked them very hard at this point. Their love, their care and support were invaluable to me — it was so reassuring to have such love around me.

During transition the most amazing thing happened. I had already reached the point of realising there was no way out of this — that I should just go with the flow — and that's exactly what I did. I found my astral body for the first time in my life and seemed to be up on the ceiling looking down on the birth of my baby. In no time, Leah was born with absolutely no drama, horror, or anything other than a few stitches — she had a relatively large head for her tiny weight of 2.5kg.

Leah is now ten years old — almost every day I flash back to the beauty of her birth and her being.

I still had to deal with my cervical cancer. I followed this up about six weeks after the birth. No trace could be found. Whilst this was very mysterious it was also a relief.

Jake was born two-and-a-half years later in a different hospital. We were living in North Queensland at this stage. Once again, a very peaceful pregnancy. This time, I came into labour ten days early and in much the same way as the first. We went off to hospital and within one hour Jake was born. I must say that this time too, the doctor I had been consulting was out of town — once again a complete stranger to contend with in my most intimate moment — but once again a very pleasant, helpful man who just seemed to be there in case he was needed.

It was wonderful having David there. His knowledge was an added bonus. I think he found it very different being 'up the other end'. It was very necessary for me to have him there — I think it's a special moment you can never experience in any other way. It did occur to me it would be good for him to experience the expectant father's position. Naturally Jake's birth gave me as much pleasure as Leah's — so now I have two beautiful births and children to reflect on.

I was very lucky in that both the hospitals I chose were small, progressive-thinking and in no way insisted on interfering with my methods.

A most important point that doctor's don't tend to emphasise is the one of 'going with the flow'. The realisation that you can't change a thing that's happening — that your body is in full control and knows what it's doing is most important. Usually, once you relax into this frame of mind, it all seems to proceed without a hitch. Fear can tend to slow down the flow and can often cause obstructions resulting in highly technical birthing interference. The mind is extremely powerful.

Having accompanied David on a number of home births over the years, I sometimes wish I had decided otherwise. The feeling of love and high emotion is differently expressed in a hospital environment.

I also accompanied David on his visit to Dr Michel Odent in

Pithiviers, France where David was inspired by mothers-to-be labouring in water. To witness the difference in labouring was wonderful.

A couple of years after Jake's birth, a routine pap smear showed a positive result once again. This time it was dealt with immediately. An explanation I received was when smears are taken, they are not always taken from the affected area. As I had consulted two different doctors, it was obvious that they had taken the smears from two different parts of my cervix. In other words the condition hadn't mysteriously disappeared after Leah's birth. Luckily, not too many years had passed by before its presence was once again detected. Another good reason for regular pap smears!

Today, Jake and Leah are seven and ten respectively. These years would have to have been the best of my life so far — motherhood is the most fulfilling and rewarding commitment that a woman can undertake. Of course we cannot expect that every day will be wonderful — children have their ups and downs too, after all they are only human. The joy they bring outweighs everything else. I find just looking at them can bring me the greatest pleasure! To all mothers-to-be, I wish you a peaceful, joyous birth and many years of sheer pleasure ahead.

And a footnote: I really sympathise with Nean's dilemma over the pap smear and the prospect of surgery. I still wonder whether pap smears ought to be performed routinely in pregnancy rather than in the post-natal period. It seems to me an unnecessary burden for a woman to have to face a decision on cervix surgery during pregnancy. Surely the overall survival rate would not be vastly different if the smear were done some six months later.

THE STORIES

Because this is what I do, people always ask me what's so good about home birth. After all these years, there are all sorts of things I can tell them, but I can really do no better than to recount any one of a number of wonderful birth experiences. They're not always easy, never the same. And the best way to really feel the power of the event is to listen to the stories of the women themselves.

THE BIRTH TEAM

Our birth team has had various helpers, midwives and doctors in attendance through the years. Over this time three women, Sister Lorna Mead, Pam Sonia and Jude Holland, stand out for their consistency and dedication to labouring women and their gentle caring approach to unborn and newborn babies.

I would have to say that Pam and Jude are as different as chalk and cheese. Jude is the epitome of the all generous earth mother, loving, emotional, intuitive and not too technical. She loves playing with babies. Pam is equally caring. She is young, efficient, sharp and intelligent. She can interpret for me the woman's wishes and help me when I forget things.

It's interesting to see how pregnant women have differing needs in their helpers and tend to gravitate naturally to one. As a woman said to me, 'I really don't need my mother at my birth', whereas another can't do without her.

The woman's support, her rod and staff indeed, can and should be her familiar midwife or a close knowing female companion, to stay with her through the long hours of labour and beyond.

BIRTH AT HOME

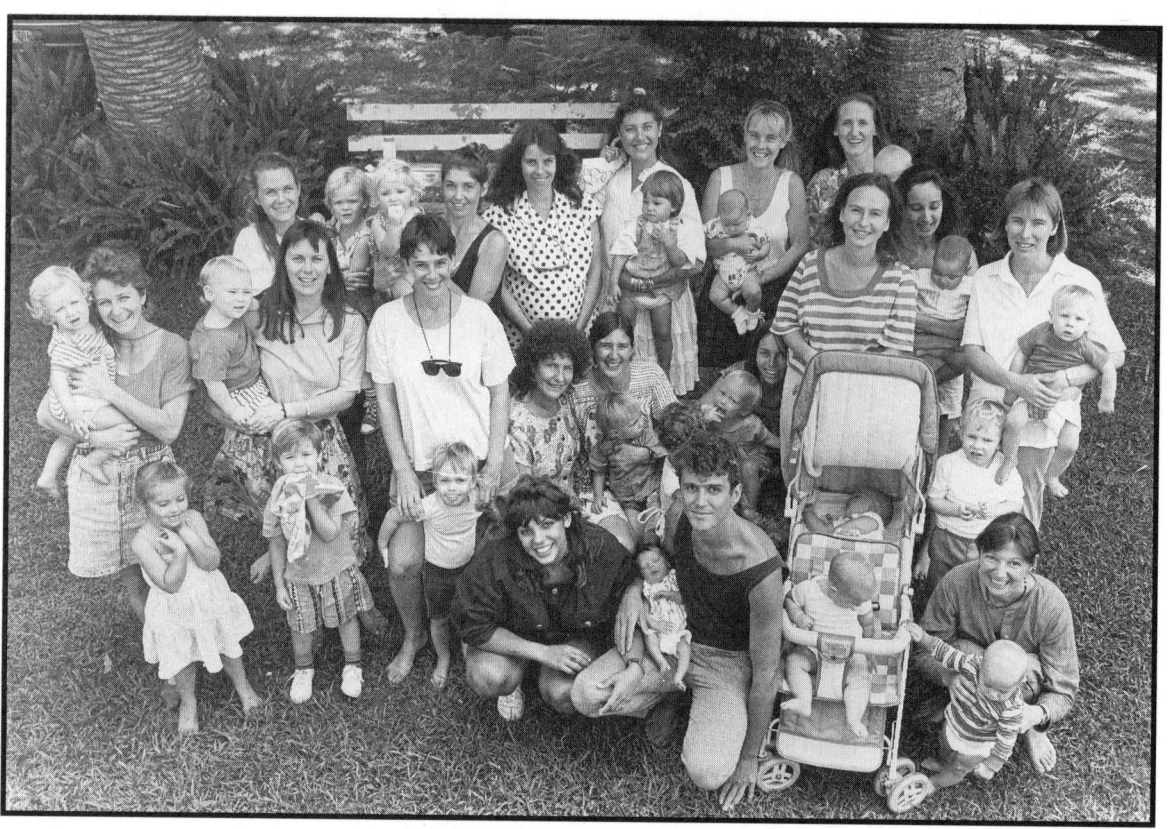

The Home Birth support group (Pam and Jude, midwives, at centre).

Home Births

A woman in labour is usually in a different space and the memory of the pain is often distorted. Describing the sensation of labour must be like describing how to ride a bike. Powerful contractions, which are out of the woman's control, often hurt, sometimes a lot. Women labour in all sorts of places. One chose the kitchen bench to lean against, rocking backwards and forwards chanting 'Why!' 'Why!' 'Why'! with every contraction. The one who is there and sees it best is the midwife. She has to support, encourage, breathe with, comfort the woman through each contraction. Some woman stay in one place, but others like to move around and the midwife has to follow her, with all the necessary bits and pieces of labour, as handmaiden.

David Miller

BIRTH AT HOME

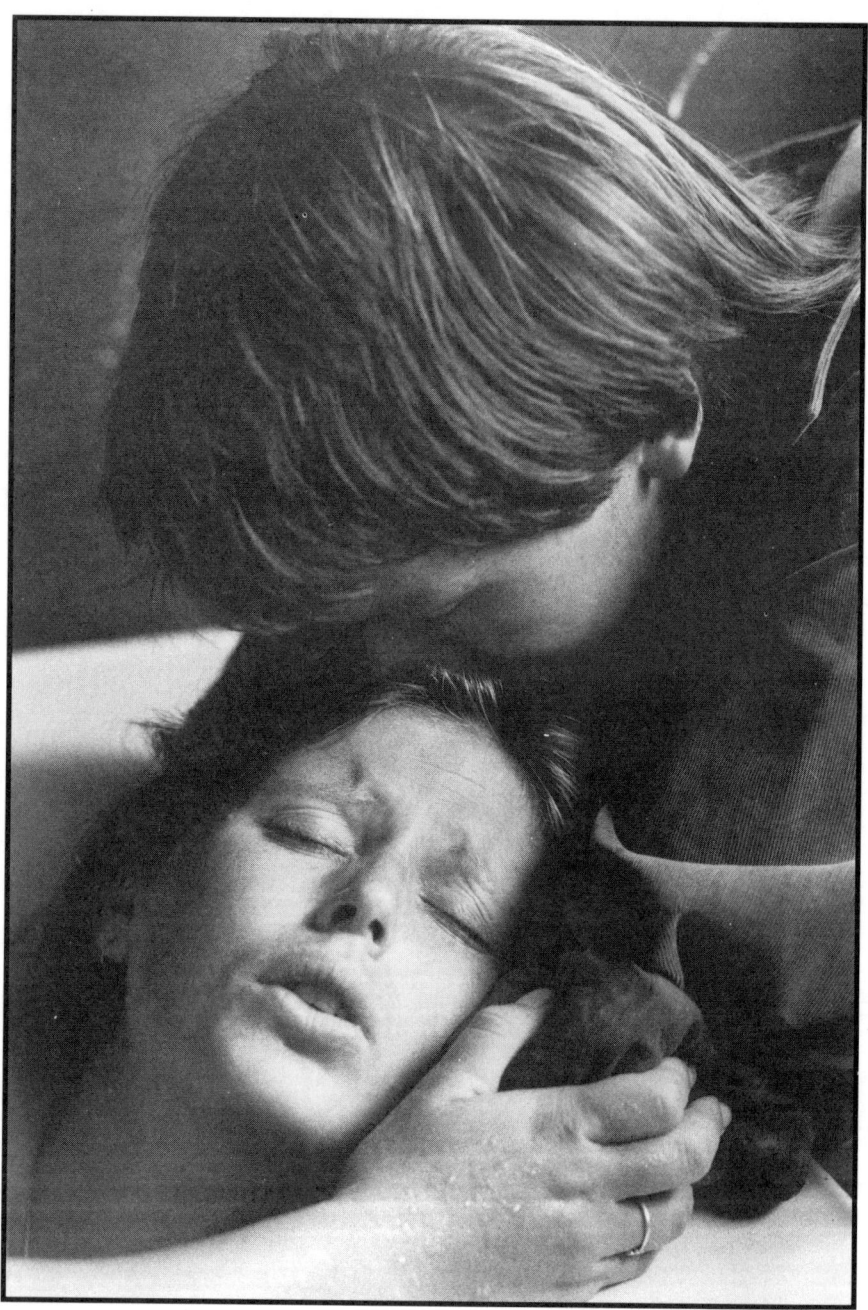

HOME BIRTHS

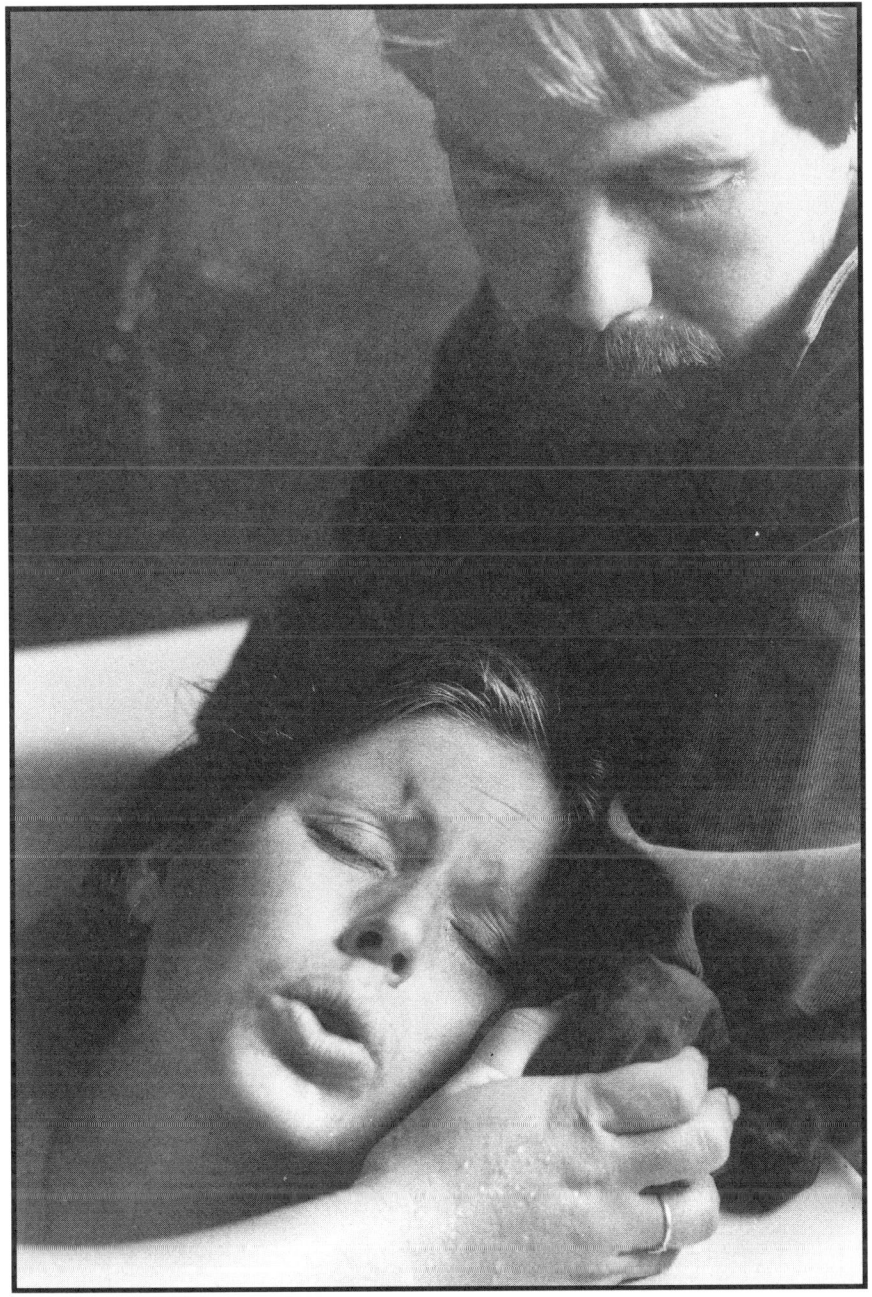

BIRTH AT HOME

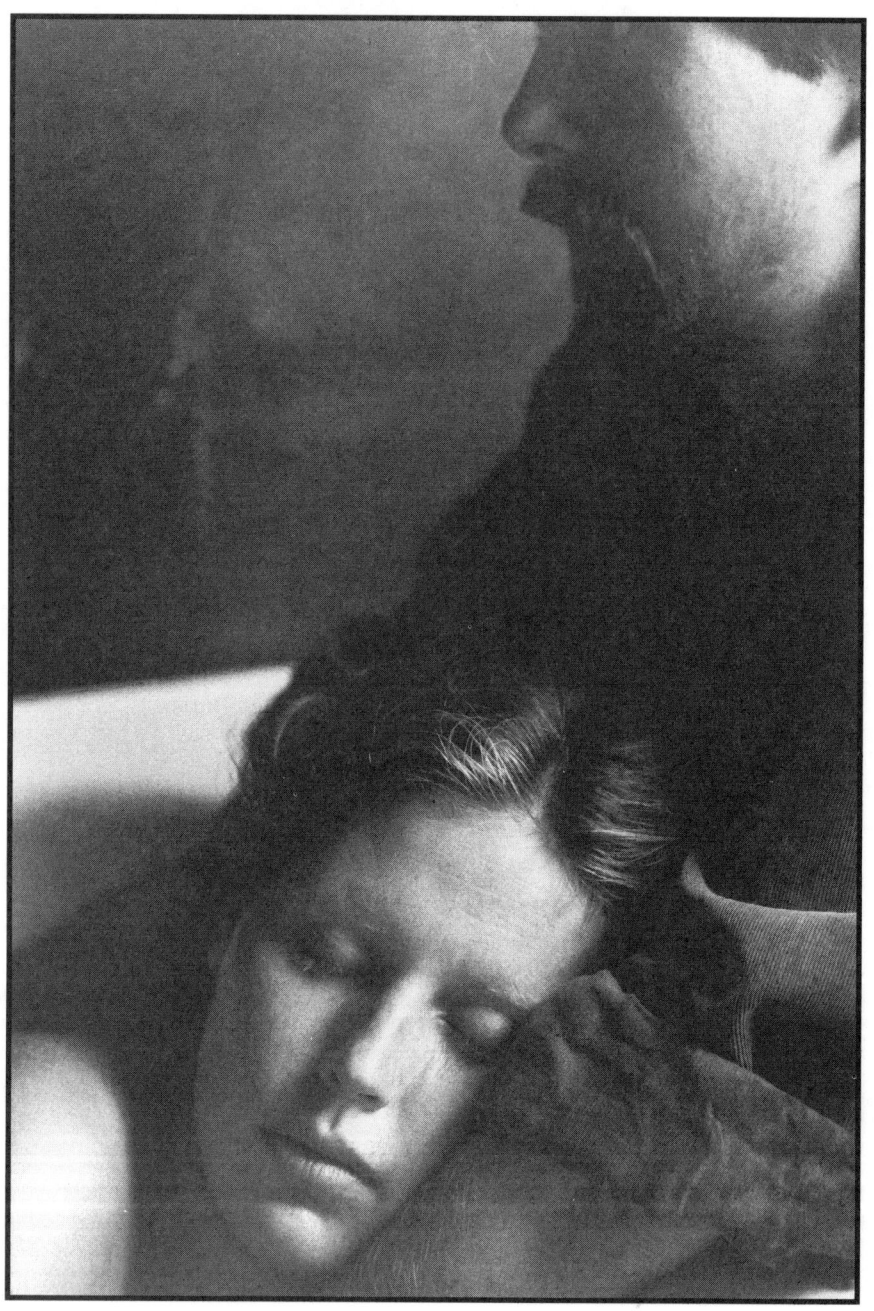

HOME BIRTHS

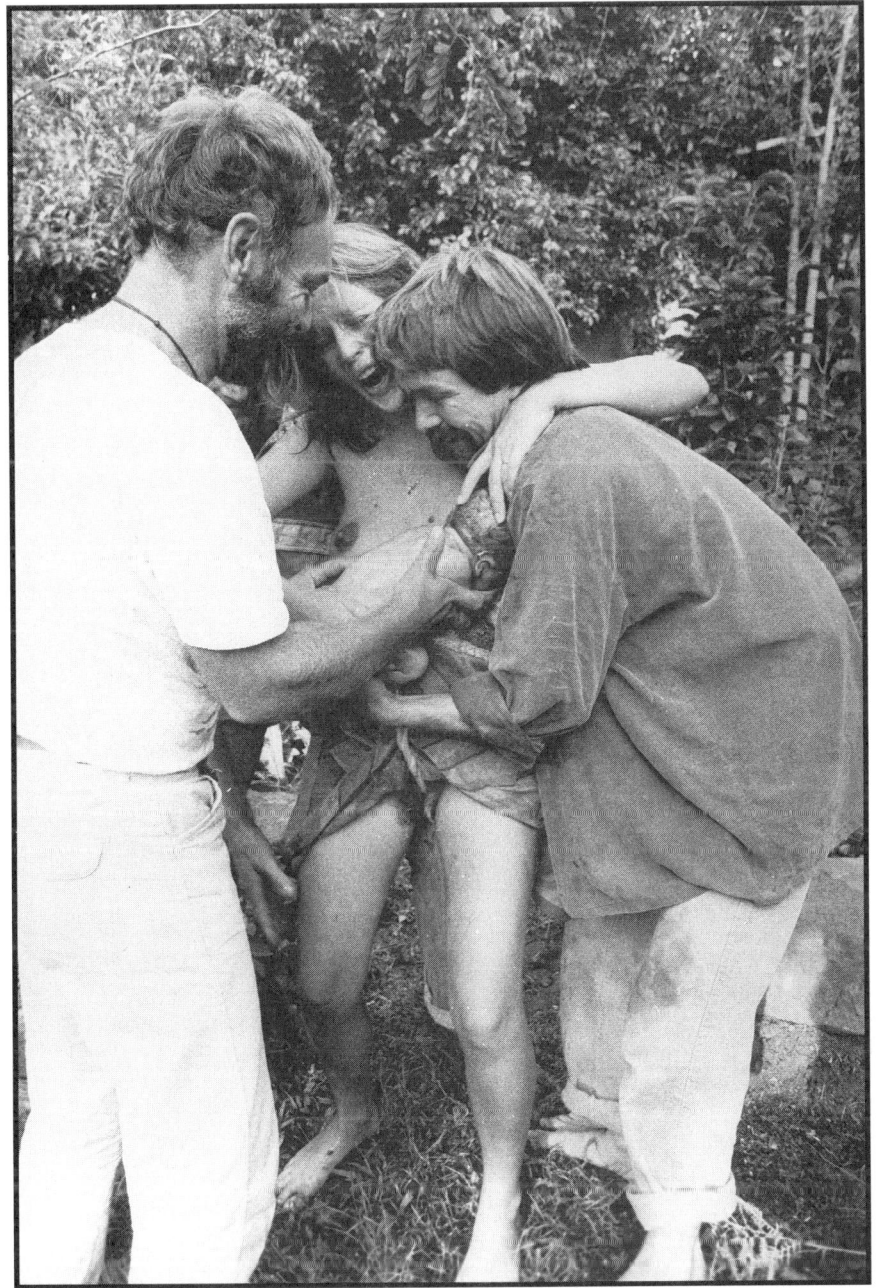

BIRTH AT HOME

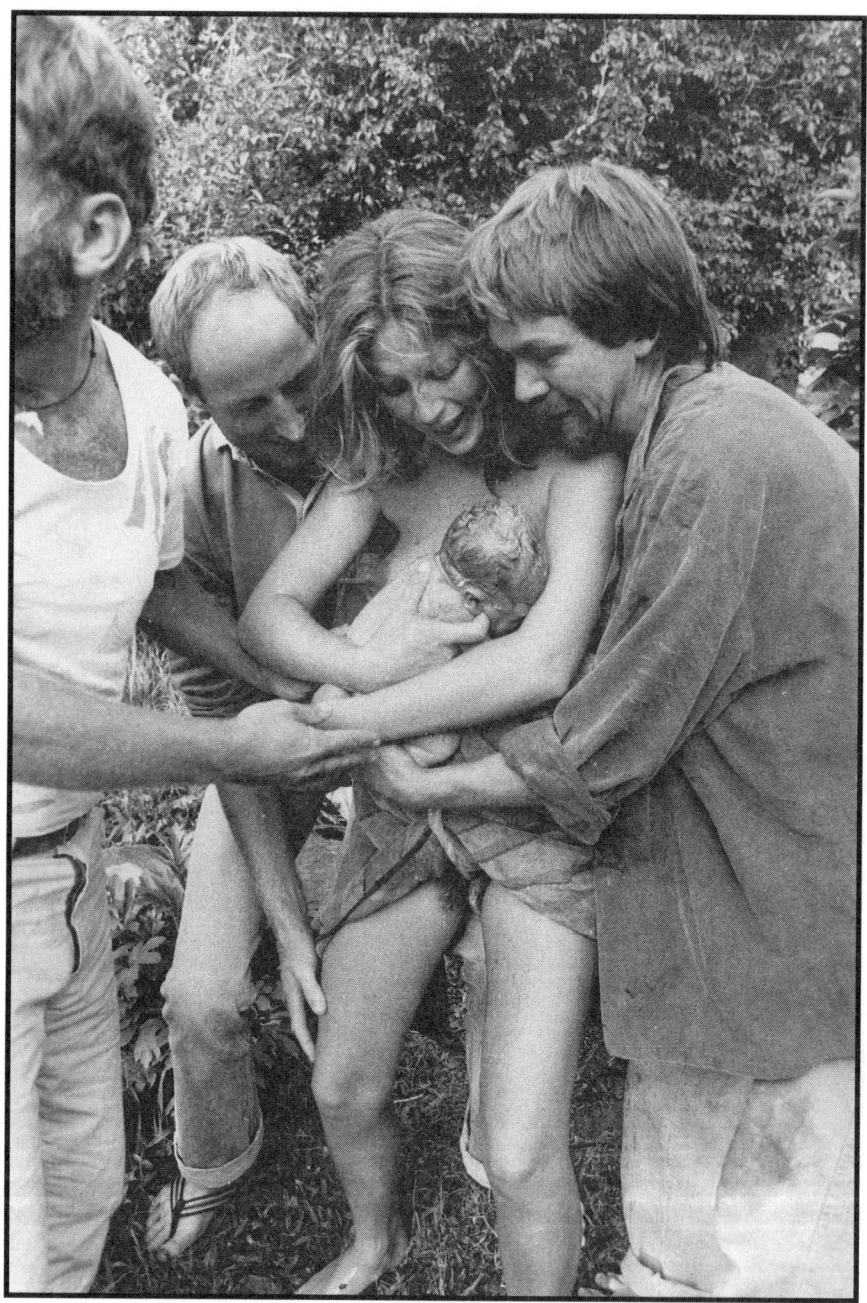

HOME BIRTHS

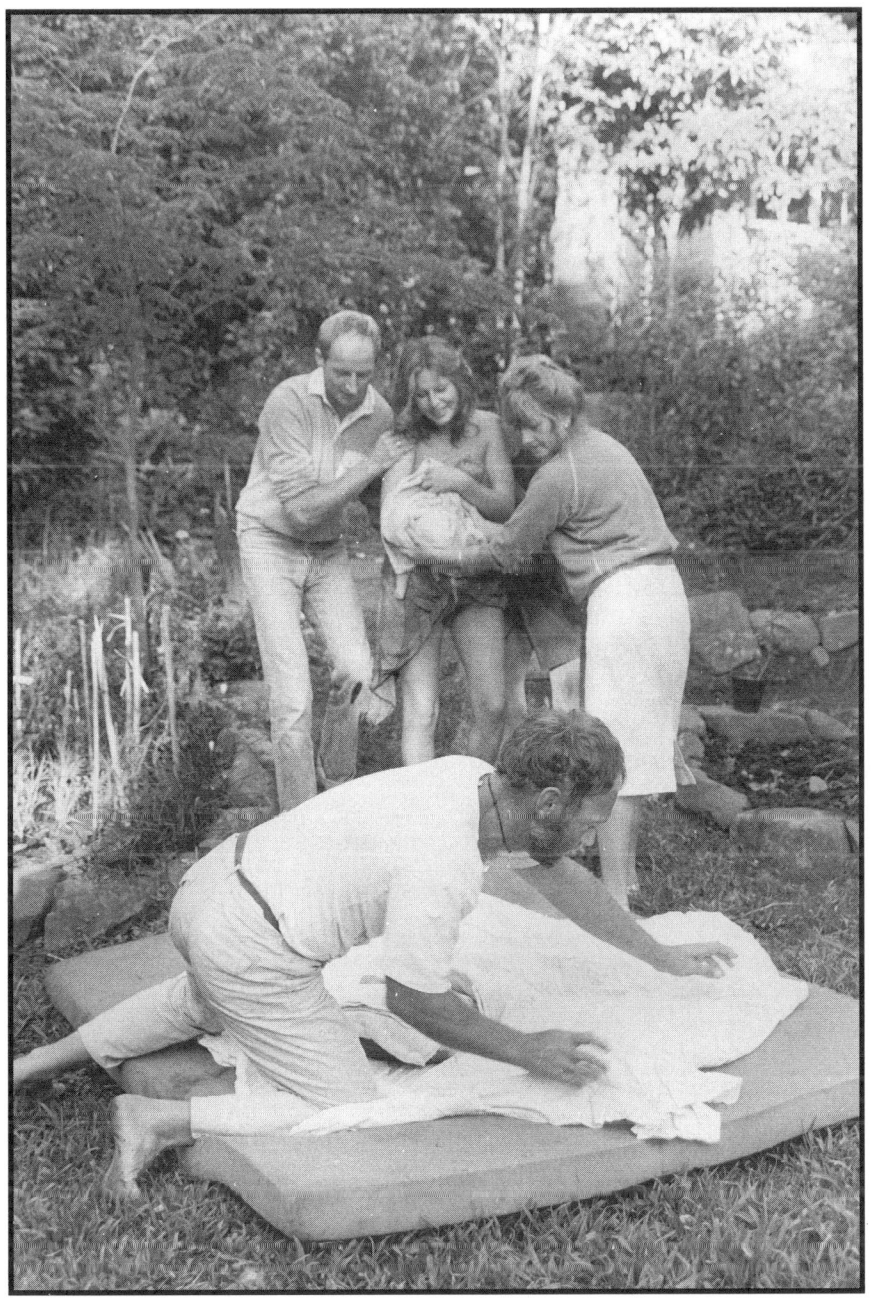

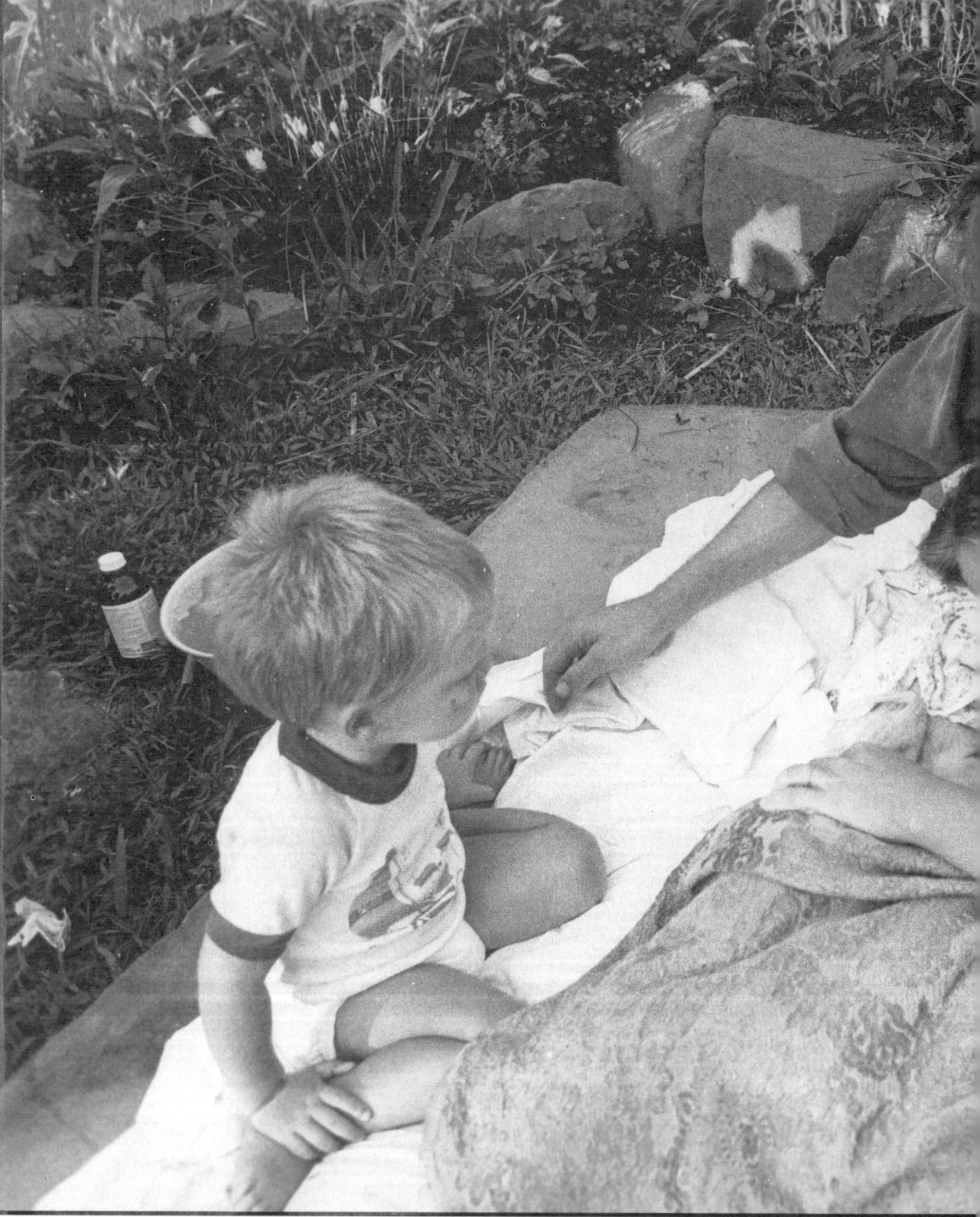

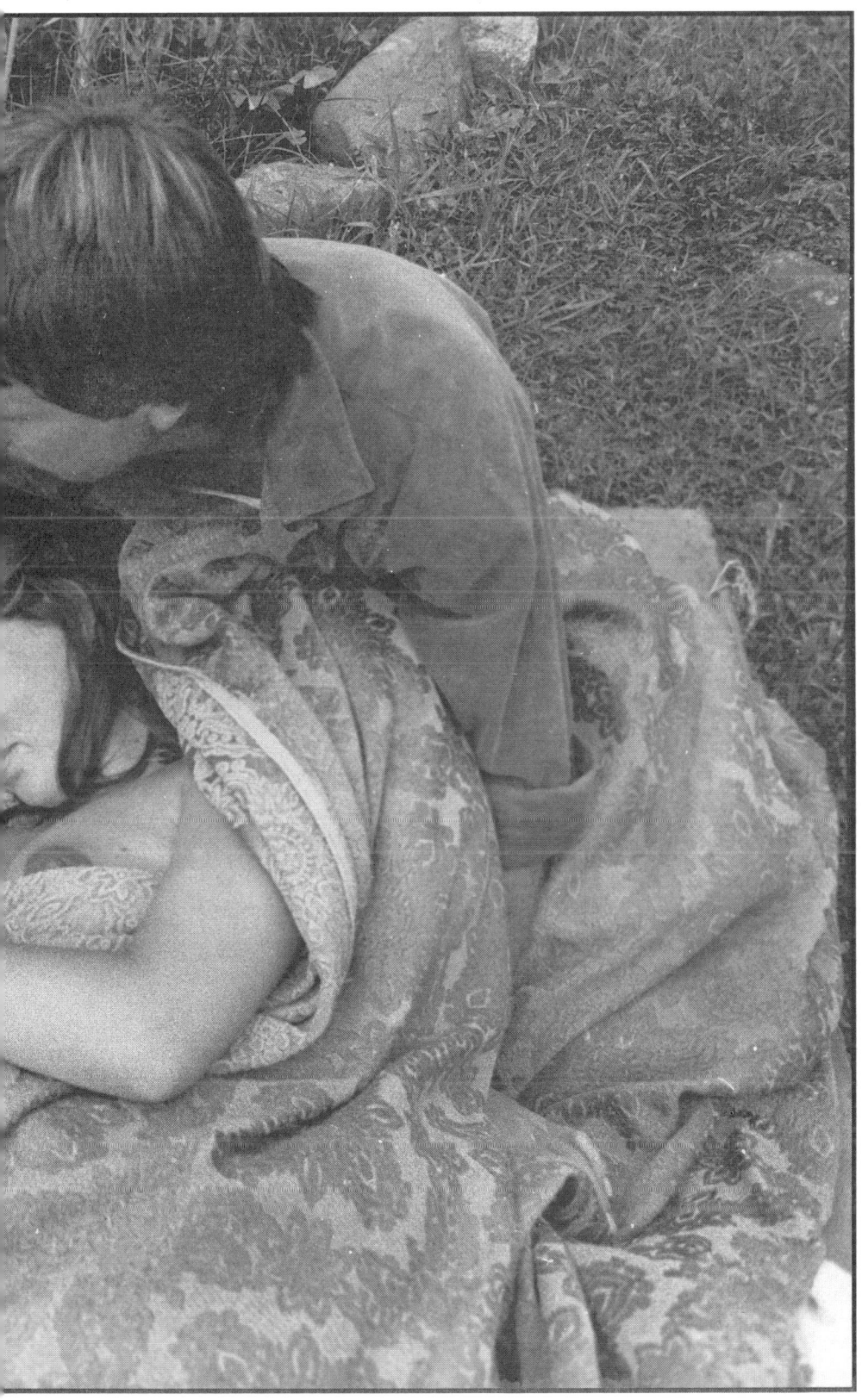

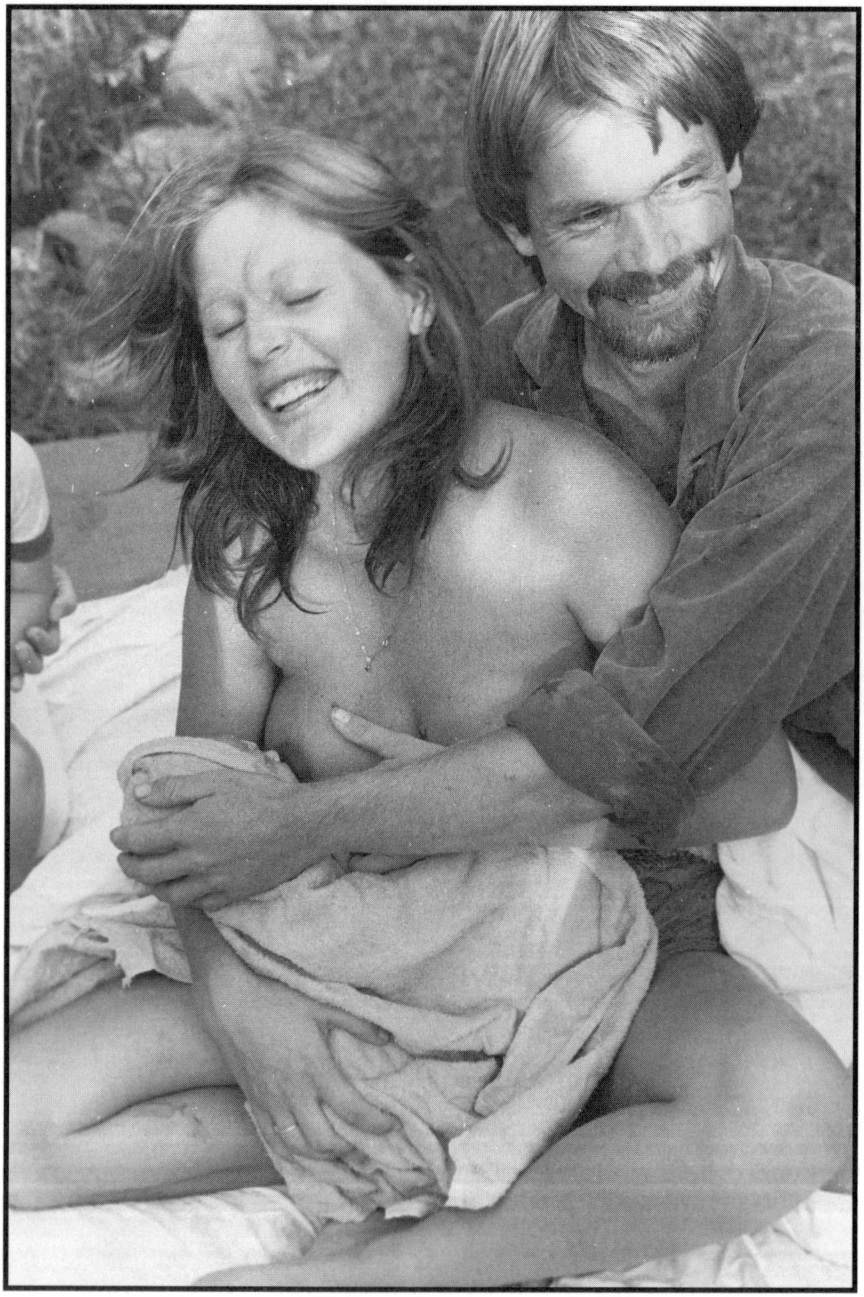

BIRTH AT HOME

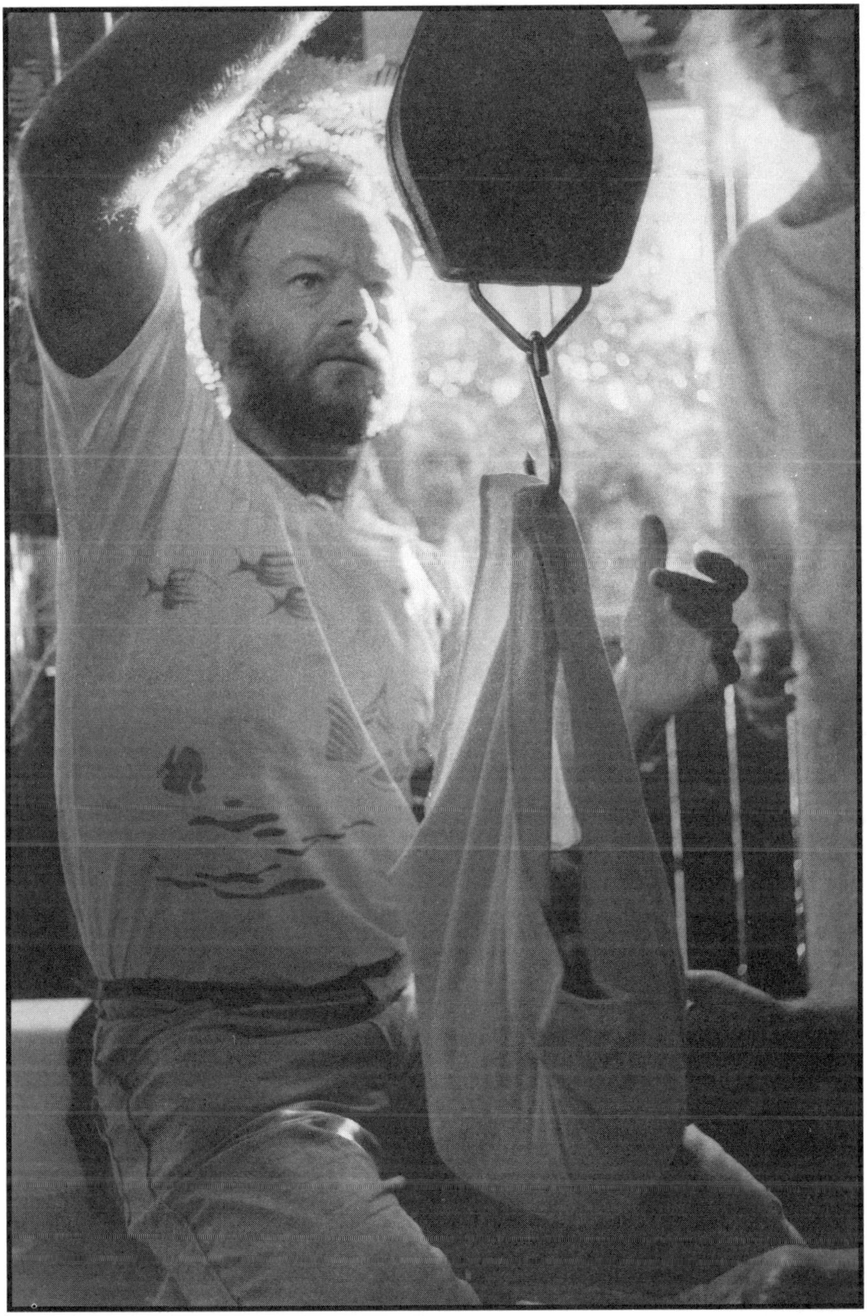

HOME BIRTHS

> *When I first began working with David I was amazed by his caring calmness and his gentle non-intervention with the mother and babe. This was extremely different from the cold sterility of the labour ward and staff at hospital. I had never seen a doctor actually comforting and supporting a labouring mum with such dedication and confidence.*
>
> JUDE, MIDWIFE

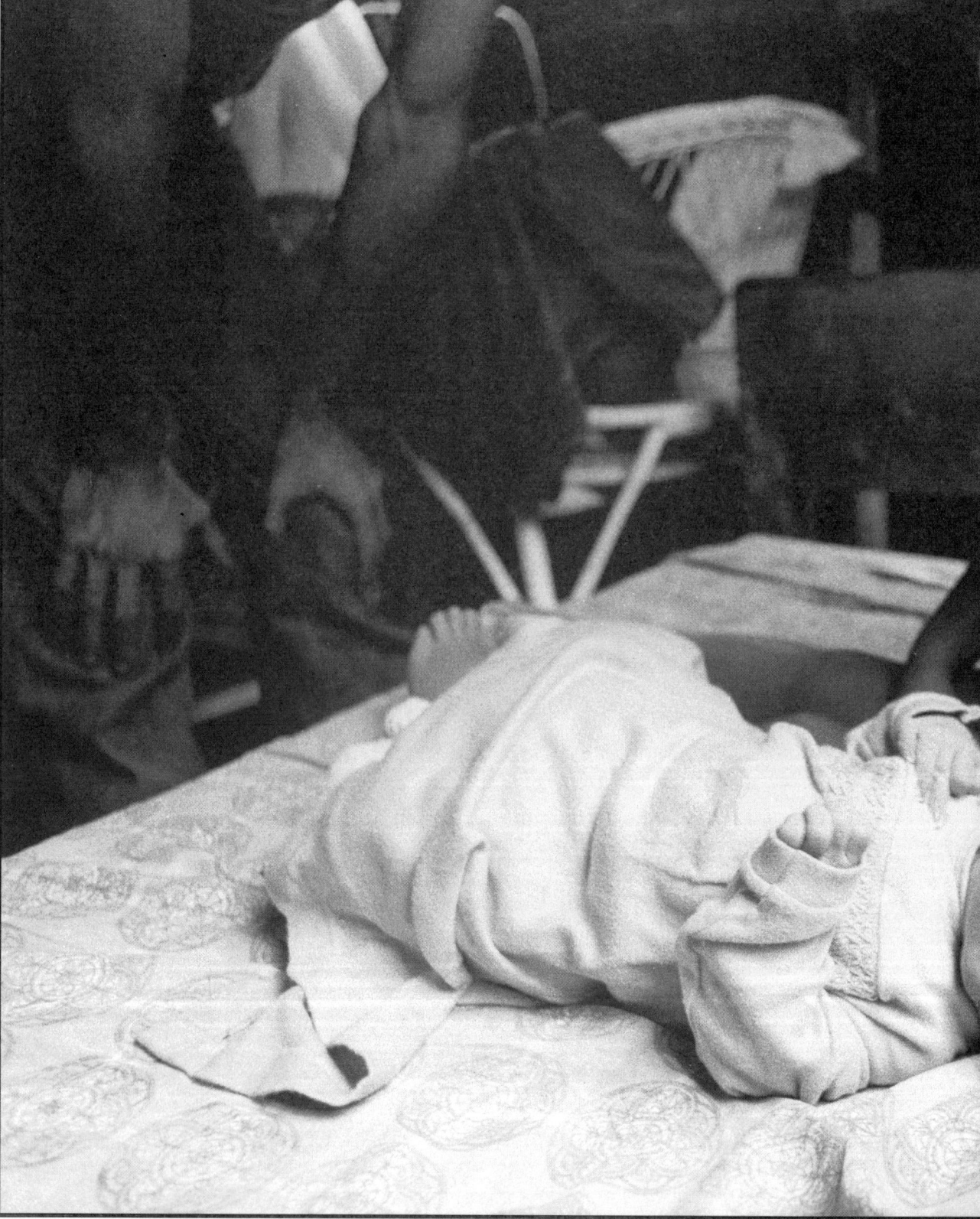

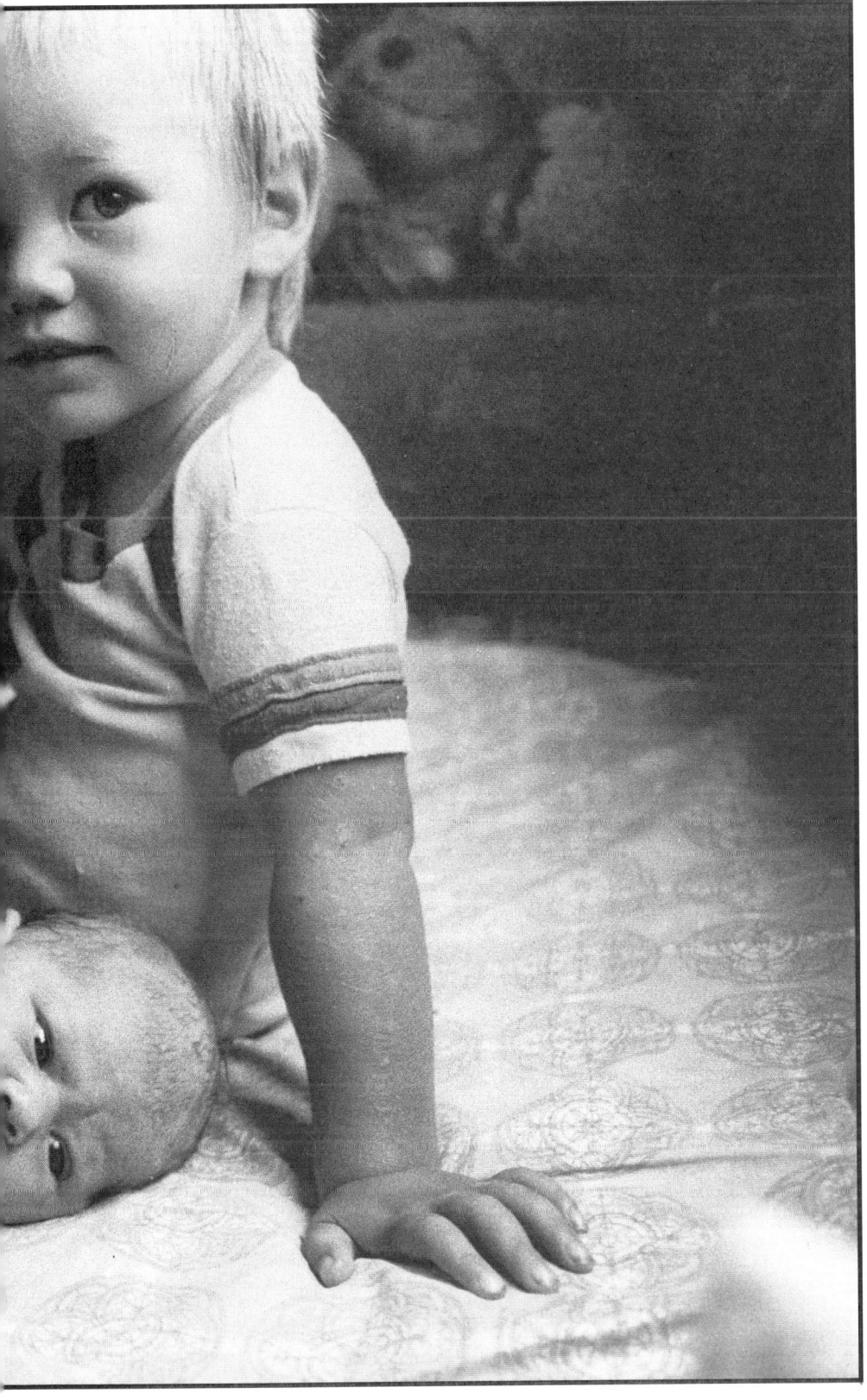

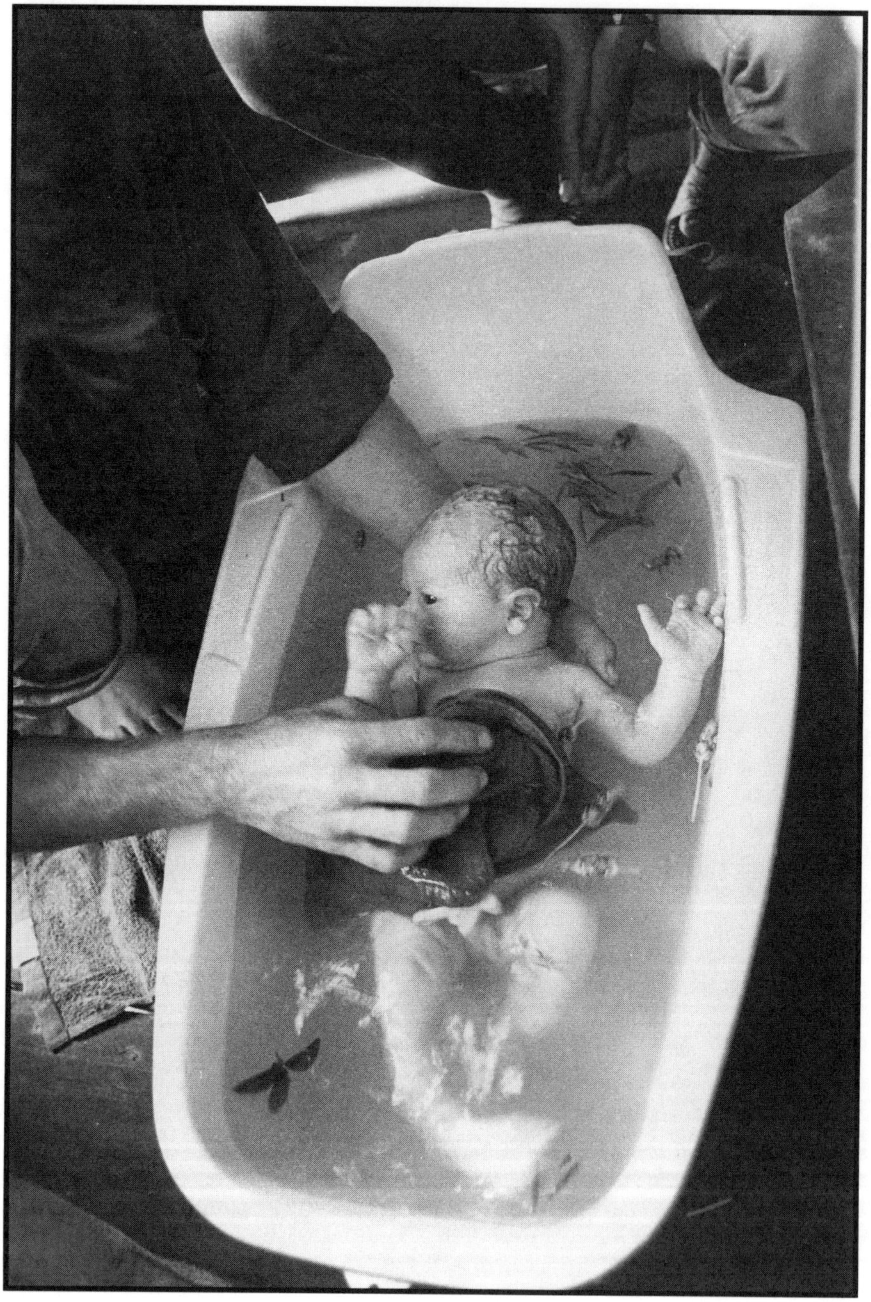

My first home birth: To Graham and Sylvia a son, Billie

The whole home birth story for me began in 1979, with Sylvia sitting in my consulting room. 'I'd like to have this baby at home,' she said. 'The others have been so easy.'

I was immediately apprehensive and clearly remember going on the defensive. 'You never know when something might go wrong,' I advised her, 'and the hospital has all the facilities.'

But she was very determined. 'This will be my last baby and Graham would like it,' she said firmly.

Graham and Sylvia were old friends, and true, their last baby, Jade, and their first delivered by me in 1976 at the local hospital had given no problems. So I agreed and set about making a list of all the things (usually found in the hospital) I might need. Making it all portable was quite a challenge. However, technology helped. Modern resuscitation and monitoring devices can be very compact. Eventually everything that might be needed fitted into three bags.

Shortly before the due date, the midwife Lorna and I drove our way up the long, steep road to visit Sylvia's house in Sun Valley. Visiting the home prior to the birth proved to be a very informative exercise. We spent time planning the possible labour scenarios, checking resources (water, heating, helping hands, child minding) communications and evacuation arrangements.

The ante natal visit has become a basic part of our home birth procedure: we check the house, its access and facilities, as well as the family situation so we are ready for any contingency, day or night.

When the big day came, we were very nervous about this step into the wild and indeed the labour was quite suspenseful and drawn out (probably as a result of our anxiety). However, we were rewarded for our patience with the birth experience of Billie, which was unlike any hospital birth — more of a family affair than a medical event. What a change for me — from the sterile operating room to a cosy living room full of smiling relaxed people enjoying the whole event.

Sylvia's Story

My fear of hospitals stems back to when I had my first son Jason in 1969. He was born in a large hospital and I had never felt so alone and scared in my whole life. I was left to labour all by myself without any support from anyone — husbands weren't allowed in labour wards in those days.

This experience left quite a scar and I was five months pregnant with my second son before I was seen by a doctor. This was when I first met Dr David in 1975 and he emphasised how important it was for me to have regular check-ups. As he was moving to the area I decided to put my trust in him — a trust he has never let down. I told him of my fear of hospitals and he assured me that Graham would be able to be with me during this birth. He did have to fight the establishment over this, and Graham was the first husband allowed in the labour ward. My second birth certainly was a lot more pleasant and I'm sure it was because Graham and David were there for support.

In 1979, when I fell pregnant the third time, Graham and I decided that this would be our last child, and it be great if we could have it at home. I approached David about it at my next consultation and he was very apprehensive, letting me know that complications do occur and that the hospital had all the facilities. I was quite determined that my last baby would be born at home and finally David relented and we set about organising a list of things usually found in a hospital that David might need.

I started labour on Saturday and being at home I was able to go about my normal routine without too much difficulty. I'm sure this took my mind off the discomfort. By late Saturday afternoon Lorna, my friend and midwife, arrived. We all sat around having dinner, joking and laughing.

Realising nothing too much was going to happen we bedded down for the night. By morning my labour pains really started happening and it was great to be at home with the kids and have Graham for moral support. As it happened, a few of my friends turned up to visit (not realising what was going on). Not only were they good company for me but they helped in the kitchen making endless cups of tea for us all.

As the time for the actual birth arrived I was surrounded by family and friends and the energy that was given to me by all of them was incredible. Every breath and push I did, they did with me, which really gave me the surge of energy I needed.

Not only did my two sons see the arrival of their baby brother (an experience they still talk about), but I was able to share this wonderful experience with Graham and my friends in the comfort of my home.

Elsbeth's baby: home birth after a caesarian

I think Elsbeth's story stands out for one important reason. The story involves the contrast between a hospital birth involving a caesarian section and a home birth, which despite her previous experience and fears was safe. Even though she'd had both a caesarian and an ectopic pregnancy (pregnancy in the fallopian tube) she presented so favourably at the end of her pregnancy that I decided it was safe to comply with her choice and go ahead with a home birth. (Of course, the final okay for a home birth to proceed is always a late decision, depending on how the pregnancy is progressing.) With Elsbeth, it was particularly satisfying to help her have a positive birth experience. It was a great victory for everyone involved and a healing for Elsbeth herself.

Elsbeth's Story — The Birth of Sam

The gynaecologist recommends a caesarian section. The baby has returned to a breech position following an attempt by the doctor to turn it around. An X-ray reveals my pelvis is 10.4cm wide and should be at least 11.6cm for a quick delivery without complications. What a disappointment after weeks of practising for a natural birth, breathing and panting my way through childbirth education lessons together with my husband. Well before the baby was due, I was to go to hospital.

It was Friday 19 May, I was nervous and apprehensive, as this was the first time back in a hospital after a tonsillectomy had gone wrong and I had to stay in hospital for two weeks, at the age of ten. At about 10.00 pm, I just had my last cup of tea and a biscuit when there was an uproar. One of the expectant mothers, a Greek woman who couldn't speak any English, was yelling. Apparently her water broke and she had been in labour for a few hours without telling the nurses. Panic reigned as she was supposed to have a caesarian and within thirty minutes everything had to be prepared for the operation.

After all the commotion I was so tense I had to be given a sleeping tablet. In the morning the nurse came to take a blood sample — nothing to eat, two laxative suppositories, which did their job $1\frac{1}{2}$ hours later, I felt quite ill. Then came the dressing-up part with a sterile gown, leggins and a hat, and then a catheter was inserted. Soon I was to have an epidural, there were several students present watching the proceedings, but I didn't mind.

For the epidural you have to roll yourself up like a cat so that the anaesthestist can place the injection between the vertebrae. I could feel the effect of the anaesthetic numbing my legs, suddenly I felt nauseous and very dizzy, my blood pressure dropped and there was a slight panic, but it soon passed and I was glad to be awake for the event. I didn't feel any pain, just a tugging and pulling and I could feel my tummy lighten as the baby was lifted out. It was a cute little bundle — a baby boy. He was a bit blue and had to be given oxygen. When he recovered, my husband, who was present, gave him a Leboyer bath. At that time the Queen Victoria was one of the few Melbourne Hospitals open to Leboyer techniques, and demand feeding and rooming-in were encouraged.

Birth of Joni

Seven years later I was pregnant again. It was quite a surprise because five years earlier I had an ectopic pregnancy and one of my

BIRTH AT HOME

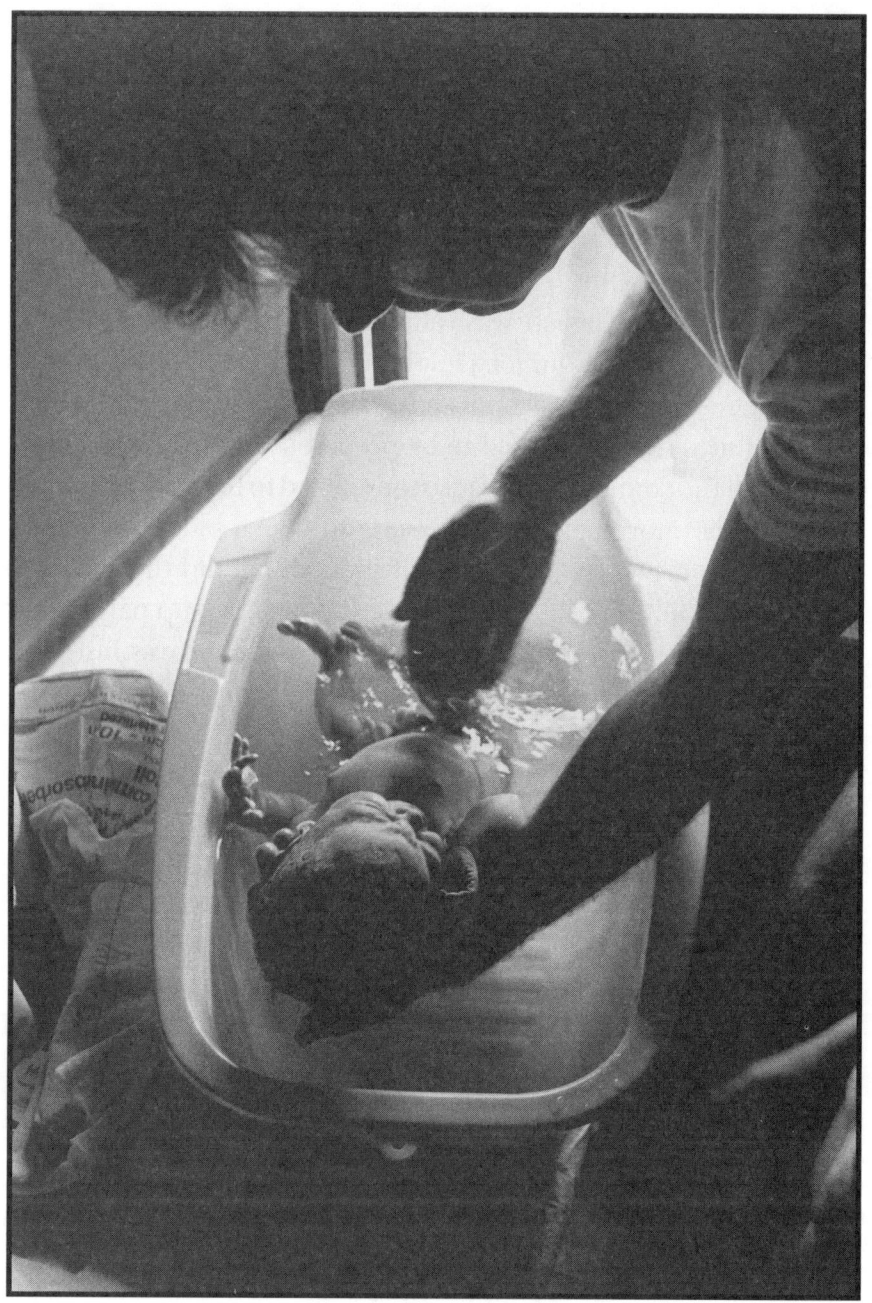

HOME BIRTHS

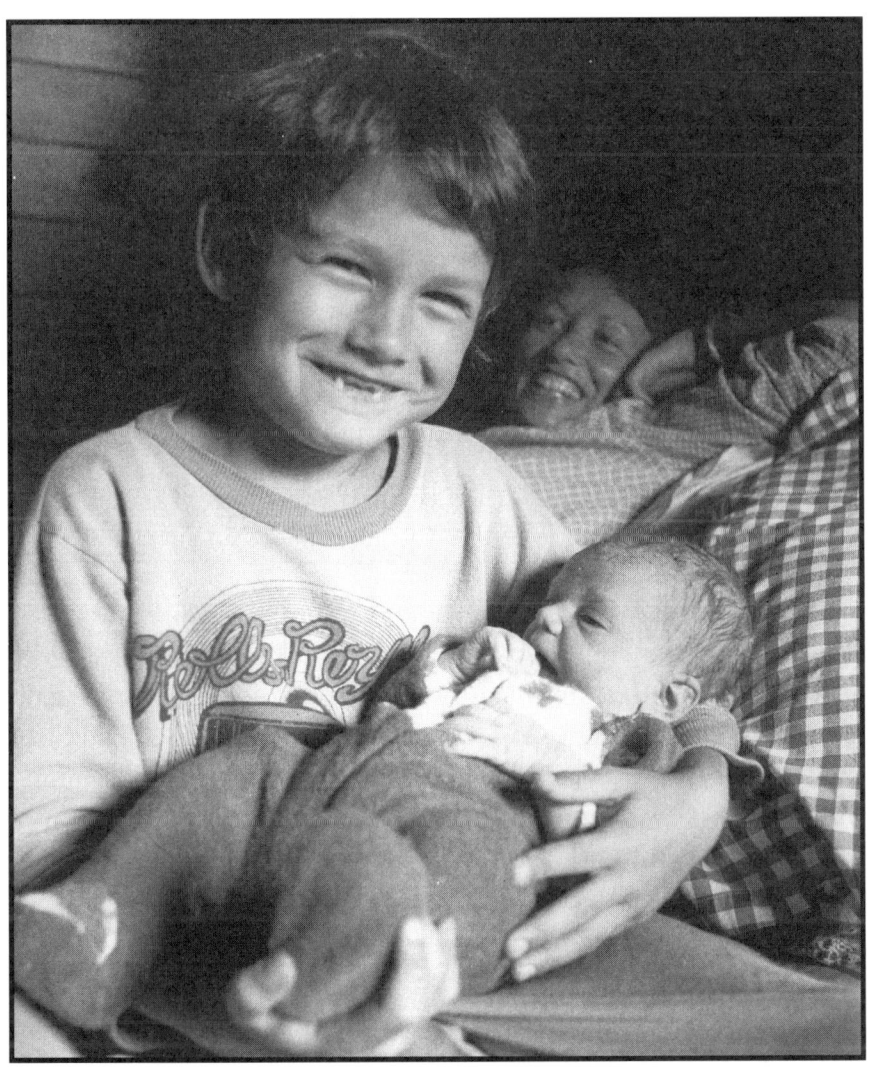

fallopian tubes had been removed, supposedly reducing the chances of conception. There seemed to be no major problems during the pregnancy and although I had been advised by the Melbourne specialist to have future births by caesarian section, I was determined to have a natural birth this time and, if possible, at home.

I was lucky to have Dr David Miller as my obstetrician. He was specialising in home births. He was encouraging and we had a good understanding throughout the ante natal care. A minor bleeding called for an ultrasound examination towards the end of pregnancy and I also had some acupuncture to help the baby's head engage. The baby was not in a breech position this time.

It was midnight. I was still awake and a strange excited feeling had taken hold of me and prevented me from sleeping, and as I turned over my water broke and soon after, the first wave of a contraction was tightening my tummy.

We got busy changing the sheets and getting everything prepared for the birth. We rang David Miller to let him know that things were on their way. Comfortable in my bed we tried to get some more sleep before it all got too hectic. At 4.00 pm David arrived with the midwife and some of my friends. By that time the contractions were coming and going and David was pleased with the progress.

I sat in a warm bath for a while, but felt safer back in my bed because I seemed to want to totally relax from my waist down, as not to block any openings and to let the force of the contractions do their work. The scar of the previous operation never bothered me. It was now about 7.00 am in the morning. I could hear a kookaburra laughing, it was a beautiful sunny morning as the little baby girl greeted the light of day. Six hours of labour.

Having an understanding doctor, a kind midwife, my husband, my mother, my seven-year-old son, and some of my friends with me was, for me, the best way of bringing a brand new person into this world. Even for my mother it was a great experience. She sat down and wrote a five page letter to my family in Switzerland.

HOME BIRTHS

Violet: born in the garden. Why not?

Julie is a dynamic and spontaneous woman. This really came out in the labour. We (the support team) had to move very quickly to keep up with this sprite. You had to be fit — up and down the ladder from her bedroom, out to the garden, into the bath house, out again — and the unexpected delivery with Julie standing on a rock step in the path. I've never seen John McCormick move so fast with his camera gear. His series of photographs of Violet's birth are included, because they so beautifully supplement Julie's story.

I still shudder slightly when I read Julie's account of having to be moved from the bath she was enjoying to go inside for the birth. At the time of this birth, the team had as yet no experience of actual birth in water, which I later came to see as a viable choice. These days, she would probably stay in the bath. Anyway, at least we were flexible enough to stop on the path when she said the baby was coming and let her have her baby in the garden. It was a beautiful day, after all.

Julie's Story

Violet, my second child, was born at home on 17 January, 1985. My birthing team being David, my doctor; Lorna, his assisting midwife;

Jude, my dear friend; Michael, my acupuncturist; John, our photographer; and of course my main support, my husband Eric. A week before Violet was due David came to our mountain home for his routine 'before birth visit' to familiarise himself with our surroundings and to make sure all was in order. We were planning to have the baby in our loft bedroom.

My labour began on the sunny afternoon of my due date. Everyone was contacted and arrived at our home. I laboured slowly through the night, the contractions being consistent but fading off at times. I became restless towards morning and felt like being in a different space, other than my bedroom. I wanted to have a bath. Our bathroom is a separate building to the house. I was helped down our ladder and up through the garden to the bathroom. The water in the bath relaxed me and my contractions grew stronger and came faster. Before I knew it I was bearing down in the bath. I knew my baby was coming. Immediately Lorna pulled the plug from the bath. Water birthing was a new unexplored experience to my team at this stage. I was helped from the bath and was to be carried back to the house for the baby's delivery. I was thinking to myself, 'No way am I going to make it back inside.' I felt the head crowning and demanded to be put down. Instinctively, I was looking for a place to have my child out there in the garden.

David felt me as I stood there supported by Eric and Michael, and he realised I wouldn't be moving from that rock step I was standing on. (The two women were inside preparing the bed with sterile sheets etc. for the delivery.) He looked into my eyes and said, 'OK we're doing it right here, right now, standing.'

He then told me I could push. After about two pushes the head was delivered and then the body just seemed to slip out. John had his camera set up outside and only just caught the birth. Jude and Lorna came running out with a mattress and sheets to place me and the baby on. I fumbled to get my arms from around Eric's and Michael's shoulders so I could embrace my baby. I took her in my arms and tried to lift her up to kiss her but the umbilical cord stopped her, so

I had to bend down and kiss her.

The sun was just rising. I was helped to the mattress and Violet fed from my breast while the placenta was delivered. Kye, our son, awoke and came out in the garden to join us and meet his sister. There we all were up on Mt Boogarem in our garden. A truly natural birth. Violet was named after the native violets that were growing all around our house. This was to be Lorna's last birth with David and the beginning of Jude's midwifery. It could have been their first water birth but instead it was their first outdoor birth.

Lani Joy: A Grandmother's Story

The next contribution is from Joy, a grandmother who came from the city to attend her daughter Kaye during labour and the time afterwards. It's a wonderful story with such a huge cast of happy and involved players that I've decided I'd better preface it with an explanatory list of who's who.

As Joy's diary of the events illustrates, in natural birth it's not always easy to work out the time of birth in advance. I remember sitting outside around the big fire, drinking endless cups of tea with Joy. Like everyone else she wanted to know when the baby was going to come. I had to reply, 'I really don't know — we just have to wait for the baby.' I had to explain that it's easy to get anxious during these long waits — but there's no danger — and we all just had to relax.

So while Joy talks about the birth, she also talks about the events and emotions involved while waiting. Quite a saga really — the wait, in this case, was almost two weeks! It's interesting how the detail in this diary shows the feelings and the atmosphere that can be part of home birthing.

Joy's Story

Joy — Grandmother — storyteller
Hoss — Dad
Kaye — Mother

HOME BIRTHS

Ros — close friend
Pete — Kaye's brother
Jane — Pete's wife (a mother to be)
Dr Ian — Ros's husband and local G.P.
Solai — Hoss and Kaye's first-born son
Lani Joy — new baby

I've just arrived home from *Namara-Tya* with glowing warm emotions tingling in my body. The days which preceded Lani Joy's birth on 3 September at 1.01 am were filled with frustrations, happiness and, fortunately, loads of laughs.

I had set off on the bus on Tuesday evening 21 August, after we had received a call from Kaye early that morning to say contractions had started. I arrived at *Namara-Tya* some fifteen hours later, not knowing if the baby would beat me to it.

Day 1 21 August   after Kaye's phone call, I was very disappointed that I probably wouldn't make the birth. So now I was really hoping I would be around for this blessed event.

Yes, I was in time, but the contractions ceased soon after I arrived. A great anti-climax. So after soothing cuppas we all settled down for the night.

Day 2 Kaye visited Dr Miller later that morning, baby expected within two days. I was so happy to spend these waiting days with Kaye, Hoss and Solai. I always feel it is a special time for mothers and daughters just before a birth. It's not always possible to be together. We spent the next few days quietly — great to see Pete and Jane. Usual Friday visit to Dr Miller. A quick introduction, also met Pam the midwife and she seemed very warm and friendly. The baby would arrive within a week. The days dragged by — no sign of a birth. Dr Ian and Ros were marvellous and kept the days happy and relaxed when they popped in. The Kaffee Klutch was a highlight of the endless waiting. Pete's humour added a sparkle to the long days which followed.

Another week went by — I changed my bus ticket from Saturday 1 September to Tuesday 4 September — just hoping something would happen before then. The weekly visit to Dr Miller on Friday once again. He tried to stimulate the obstinate cervix, suggested Kaye go home, have a tablespoon of castor oil, a hot bath and some caullophylum — homeopathic brew — surely something would start.

Day 9 It was Friday evening 31 August, Kaye and I were frantically knitting the 'birth robe'. We purchased this beautiful ivory coloured cotton with a silk thread, in the morning. Very optimistic that we could finish in time — it did give Kaye something to think about. We didn't realise the garment was knitted in one piece 235 stitches on No. 12 needles. I copped this and Kaye the sleeves.

Solai was asleep and Hoss decided on an early night. The strain of the last eleven days was starting to tell. His tummy was in nervous conflict and he needed to be fit for the birth.

The smell from two freshly baked banana cakes was a joy to the nostrils. The aroma mingled with the strong perfume of the jasmin. Kaye had it everywhere, it's supposed to be excellent for getting labour started. All serene and a beautiful atmosphere. The reflection from the little cane shade in the kitchen cast most interesting patterns on the walls and the ceiling. A warm glow from the one fire stove and a great feeling of love from this small home.

Suddenly this peaceful haven came alive — a contraction and another one. Hoss and I sprang into Plan A, that early night was not to be. The table had to be moved against the wall — it needed skill to guide the wonky leg, Kaye and Hoss on all fours completed the job — a quaint sight. 'I might fix that leg,' said Hoss. I was relieved he didn't start the job then.

The sterilised birth bundle is placed on the freshly cleaned table top alongside the baby's clothes with piles of linen and towels. The tripod set and ready to record the home birth — this was Dr Ian's department. What a tower of strength he has been right through.

The potty placed alongside the door and the bucket and bag of sawdust all ready to cope with the enema. Sawdust I have learned is a great thing in the bush. Hoss and I made our way down the steps to the woodpile by the outside loo (the only one). The Valley looked clear and mystical, quite breathtaking — a great night for a birth. The

HOME BIRTHS

air was so fresh our cheeks tingled as we carried the logs up to the house to chop.

More contractions, every two-and-a-half minutes — only mild. One fire stove well alight and kettle in position. I felt a sense of excitement as I ran the bath for Kaye. A hip bath just outside the kitchen area, hidden by a bamboo divider and indoor plants lending a soft leafy decor beside the hurricane light.

Hoss chopped mountains of wood, the one fire stove does use a lot of fuel. He then tended to the mood music — a real hectic off beat number. Could this have caused the contractions to stop? Luckily the tape changed to a beautiful birthing tape, sounds of trickling water and flutes, very soothing. Too late — the contractions had stopped.

Kaye back to knitting. Hoss stretched out, this waiting and now a second false alarm, too much for the expectant father. Hoss had lit incense and the aroma took over from the hot cakes and jasmin. The smoke gently floated loftwards, to my bedroom. Strange how I seem to be able to tolerate incense now. I well remember my reactions in Glen Waverley.

Yes, the years could have mellowed me — here I am waiting to witness my first home birth. I returned to the birthing robe. 9.35 — at last another contraction. 11.10 things quiet — only one contraction in the last half hour.

Hoss stirred, came and sat by the fuel stove ready for a cuppa. He held his head in his hands and muttered, 'Oh God, Oh God I'll need to sleep for three days when this birth is over but I know that won't be possible.'

Well it was time for bed, another false alarm. Kaye seemed serene and calm outwardly. She must have been so frustrated. The posy of flowers looked so lovely in the kitchen. Hoss gathered the flowers near Jane and Pete's this morning. All natives, vivid colours — they just added that little extra something.

Day 10 Kaye had a good sleep. Rich roast blend and soldiers of toast all round. A beautiful morning. I set myself up with my knitting at 6.30 am — no time to lose and what a view, right down the valley —

across to the light house at Byron Bay and beyond the ocean.

10.30 am — a show. Kaye rang Dr Miller — stove alight and kettle in position. Hoss, Kaye and Solai off to wish Rob a happy birthday — Kaye decorated one of the cakes and Hoss composed a nifty verse. I kept on knitting, a touch and go finish. 12.15 — second show. Pam the midwife rang and Pete and Jane arrived with great speed. They didn't receive the correct message and expected the head to be showing — brought bag of goodies.

5.00 pm — Pete, Jane and Solai go to Rob's.

5.02 pm — Kaye started beautiful pizzas for tea.

5.20 pm — Pam rang, suggesting a walk and nipple stimulation!!

5.30 pm — Kaye, Hoss and Zoe (the dog) walked to nearby Gerry and James'.

6.15 pm — Kaye has hot bath, great plumbing job in primitive surroundings, constructed by Pete's Plumbing Service, a great luxury. Hoss has fitted the bath in superbly.

6.18 pm — Dr Ian and Ros arrive with goodies.

6.41 pm — Pete in trouble galore with tick bite.

8.00 pm — Pete organised a book on birth time $2.00 per head.

8.50 pm — Pete called for champagne — voted against. Hisses of disapproval.

9.30 pm — Pam rang. Pete took champagne top — foil only to fix Jane's car (odd I thought).

9.55 pm — all depart.

10.15 pm — Kaye bed.

10.35 pm — I'm still knitting, an all day effort. Hands are feeling the pinch.

Day 12 Sunday 3.15 am — movements below — contractions every three minutes. Rain falling on the roof above me — I awake to the axe pounding again. Hoss replenishing the wood supply and making sure the wood is out of the rain. Hoss lit the fire and the kettle is in the 'go' position.

5.00 am — enema time.

6.30 am — contractions eased off — so frustrating and the time dragging badly.

6.32 am — Jane rang.

7.45 am — the birthing robe finished — what a job. A Kaye/Joy creation.

8.30 am — Dr Miller rang — coming out to break the waters.

9.00 am — Pam arrived with a bunch of freesias — beautiful.

9.15 am — Jean, Noel and Pete rang. Hoss back in bed. Nerves are a terrible thing. A fantastic day, rain cleared and just heavenly sunshine. It's Father's Day. Hoss could have a special gift today.

9.20 am — Dr Ian and Ros arrived armed with goodies.

9.30 am — Dr Miller arrived and the breaking of the waters. No big rush — we all expected a Niagara Falls, not so.

10.30 am — Ros took morning tea orders — we all relaxed to the trickling waters and flutes on the birthing tape. Kaye relaxed out in the sun in the cane chair. Here's hoping for a rush of the waters. Dr Miller suggested a walk. Hoss suggested Ma Joy should now be called Ma Veer — an appropriate name after all the polishing I've done. Rubber gloves worn out.

11.15 am — a walk to Keith's house. Hoping to get things going. Quite a rugged walk by city slickers standards — ground very uneven, Hoss, Ros, Zoe and myself tried to set the pace for the rotund Kaye. Kaye survived the slopes and still nothing doing.

12.14 pm — champagne opened — I couldn't wait any longer — sweet — beautiful.

12.30 pm — Pete and Jane arrived with bags of goodies from the market. We pretended the birth was over. They were shocked and it was only a teddy wrapped up after all.

12.45 pm — Kaye had a bath, she looked amazingly relaxed and very suntanned in her lovely white maternity dress and little touch to the ears — violets from Ros' garden. Kaye stoked the fire thoughtfully, what a pile of wood we've been through. Mick arrived with a lovely etching of the valley — subtle pregnant lady in the foreground. Kaye was thrilled. Mick left shortly after.

Ros and Jane whipped up a great salad and we all had delicious sandwiches out in the sun. Kaye tried to rest — disturbed by friends who came to wish her well. They were going on holidays. Pam tried to show me how to crochet a little cap to match the robe — not quite the best time to learn. Jane took over — great.

2.10 pm — tried a spot of OM. This is a type of meditation. Kaye in the centre of the circle with a spray of jasmin. We all sat around her, holding hands and repeating O M M mmm...over and over. A very moving experience and I could feel strong vibes coming through my hands. We all naturally thought birth thoughts. Dr Miller rang and disturbed our meditation.

2.30 pm — foetal heartbeat hard to find with the special stethescope — cause for concern for the onlookers. Dr Ian managed to find the beat on his normal stethoscope. Tremendous relief all round. Pam rang Dr Miller.

2.35 pm — squatting and deep breathing exercises. YIPEE — a couple of contractions.

2.40 pm — Kaye had a bath.

2.42 pm — Hoss and Ian replaced the generator. Hoping to have the washing machine working in the morning. A great luxury in this area. A borrowed generator and it needed a repair. Pete took Solai for a walk. Jane crochets — looks great. Joy tries a pre-birth snooze — it's been a long day.

2.45 pm — Dr Miller arrives.

3.00 pm — could be a GO this time. Pete took Solai for another walk. Good old Pete. All a bit much for Solai perhaps. It's all happening, contractions coming every five minutes and stronger.

5.00 pm — Kaye took to the bath for about four hours. Back rubs and contractions timed.

5.30 pm — Hoss prepared beautiful vegetables and noodles for dinner. Ros made a great salad. I opened two bottles of champers — sweet, sweet nectar. Ros and Jane enjoyed them too. The boys had an odd home brew and an odd champagne. Pete and Solai built a huge bonfire — great idea — somewhere to go later on. Solai found a little frog, his face was alive with excitement. He held it between his cupped hands. Alas, probably from fright, the little frog ceased to draw breath — Solai's joy turned to tears. We could had done without this. Hoss officiated at the burial on Solai's insistance. Gerry arrived with a beautiful bunch of jasmin. I was pleased to have a talk to Dr Miller. I think he sensed I was apprehensive and he successfully calmed my fears — I liked him, an unassuming gentleman.

9.00 pm — Kaye left the bath and lay on the bed — contractions seemed easier in the bath.

9.50 pm — Dr Ian lit the kerosene heater — a chill in the air. Suddenly the flames leapt high — Dr Ian acted hastily and all was well, and our attention directed to the birth again.

10.02 pm — Kaye back in the bath. Strong labour. Dr said it would be about three more hours. We were all trying to help as best we could — back rubs, leg rubs — support during contractions. Hoss was really fantastic. He didn't leave Kaye, he must have been so weary but didn't show it.

10.45 pm — back to bed — sample of urine showed ketones — not good — honey called for. Nearly out of honey as it flowed sweetly all day in the cups of herb tea.

Pete took Gerry home to replenish stocks. Kaye looking very tired — two doses of honey and ketones improved. Pete took up position of assistant back masseur with Hoss. Hoss never left his post.

Day 13 Birthday 12.39 am — back to the bath for a very short period. Hard for Hoss and Ros to help — contractions very strong. Dr Miller measured the cervix — 8cm now. Kaye in trouble — needed to push. Dr made her wait. Another measure and all is well — 10cm. It was time.

Dr scrubbed up quickly — I phoned Sal to say it was all about to happen, she listened in as Dr carefully guided the little head, only two pushes necessary — no cuts or tears and out popped this beautiful baby.

1.01 am — Dr took 'it' in his hands — turned it over and declared 'it's a girl'. These were electric moments, the little girl was placed on Kaye's tummy, wrapped in a towel and put on the breast — the cord still attached. All very emotional. Sal in tears down the end of the line. I don't think there was a dry eye in the room. Hoss was very emotional. He had been absolutely marvellous right through, so supportive and caring and now this little darling was cuddling into Kaye. Thank God a beautiful healthy baby.

We all watched enthralled as the cord was cut and tied. The cord resembled a telephone cord, only solid — not what I expected. Then a little later the afterbirth. Much larger than I thought. Dr opened it out and examined it. Patches of dark calcium deposits indicated the baby a week or so late. Time she was born. (Hoss buried the placenta next day. Jean going to plant special tree on the site when she arrives.)

Time for kisses and hugs all round — Pete had woken Solai and he was absolutely thrilled with his little sister. Hoss bathed Lani Joy, we watched in sheer amazement at this tiny creature — she was so clean, scarcely needed a bath. Pam dressed Lani Joy, decided the birth robe could wait until tomorrow !! The bed linen changed, Kaye settled back — a job well done. Kaye looked remarkably refreshed and the beautiful colours in her kimono highlighted her glowing expression.

Out came champagne and Ros' birthing cake — delicious — we'd eaten Kaye's birthing cake during the day. Dr weighed the baby — 3kg. One by one the crew left.

Kaye settled down comfortably with her little daughter tucked into her side — Solai was sound asleep in his bed.

It had been a long and exciting day, one I shall never forget. I'm sorry Noel and Jean were not here to share it all with us. I think Pete was deeply touched by the experience. I'm sure his views on fathering will mature as from today.

Dawn was close. Hoss absolutely ecstatic, no time for sleeping. He strolled to the bonfire, his flute tucked under his arm. The whole valley was soon filled with his music. He had a story to tell the world — he had just had a daughter.

Daniel: boy in a hurry

I remember the difficulties of travel the night of Daniel's birth as there was a furious storm blowing. You could hardly see the headlight beams through the lashing rain and water was tumbling all over the roads. Tonight of all nights Jude's car was broken down and all these detours delayed our departure for the birth place. Then we were caught behind a semi-trailer grinding its tortuous way up a winding section of highway. I performed a blind Kamikaze overtake and we were released on to the open road again to arrive in very fine time!

Sue's Story

We chose home birth because we wanted our children born into a warm loving environment, an environment where we had a say in what we wanted. We could choose whatever position was comfortable to give birth. We could have the people we wanted to be there. We had the same midwife with us throughout the birth to keep the energy flowing. We could hold our newborn baby and bond with it for as long as we liked without having him or her taken away. We felt these things could not be guaranteed in a hospital situation. We would be in control, well, as much in control as you can be during a birth.

It was also a challenge for me to give birth naturally without any drugs and painkillers and to allow my body to take control and do the job it was designed to without interference. What convinced us that home birth was right was that we found David, a doctor who would deliver for me. He was our safety net. We didn't want to take any foolish risks, so at the first sign of any complications he would take us to hospital. Another important factor that enabled us to choose home birth was home care after the birth. This is very important and we were fortunate enough to have my mother look after us along with Paul (my husband), who arranged to take four weeks' annual leave.

Daniel's birth was our second home birth. All through my pregnancy with Daniel we planned to have a water birth just as we had with Amy, our first born. With Amy we had not planned a water birth. I laboured in the soothing bath and just didn't want to leave when it was time to push. So she was born in the bath ... from water to water. I felt it was such a calm and peaceful way to be born. But birthing is one thing you can never plan.

It was a very rainy Monday in July, following three gloriously sunny winter days. We thought the baby would be born the previous Friday after I awoke with a slight show. But after a few contractions that was it — much to our disappointment. We even tried long walks up steep hills. But it wasn't time.

On Monday afternoon we went for our weekly visit to the doctor's. David examined me and to our amazement I was 2cm dilated without contractions. It was 5.00 pm. On reflection I thought I felt some twinges like contractions earlier in the afternoon but thought nothing of them. I also had a feeling that things would happen this night, but ignored this feeling as I did not want to get excited only to be disappointed again. It pays to heed your intuition.

On the way home I had my first contraction. Mild contractions continued six to ten minutes apart and lasted a couple of seconds until 8.30 pm when I had a show and the contractions came stronger and longer. By 9.15 pm they were every five minutes and lasting about 30 seconds. I laboured in the bedroom, kneeling beside the bed, rising up during a contraction and rotating my pelvis and resting between contractions with my head on pillows and almost going to sleep, while my husband Paul slept on the other side of the bed. Around 10.00 pm the contractions became more intense — every two minutes and lasting 30-45 seconds. So I rang Jude at 10.15 pm. She said she would ring David and then they would come.

David had to travel to New Brighton from Brunswick Heads to pick up Jude and then to Mullumbimby to pick up his things and then to our place in the pouring rain (it took them an hour to arrive).

It was just before 11.00 pm when I told Paul that I felt very 'spaced out' and went and sat on the toilet which felt very comfortable. I had a few contractions and Paul asked me if I wanted to get off. I told him I was very comfortable but thought I had better go back to the bedroom. It was just as well I listened to my intuition. With the next contraction my waters broke and I told Paul I wanted to push.

'You can't,' he said.

'I can't help it,' I cried.

The next thing I knew the baby's head crowned and I was crying to Paul to ring Jude again to make sure they were on their way, as he was trying to get my clothes off. He was then running around trying to get some towels to put on the carpet. Just then we heard David and Jude pull up. I felt so relieved to know they were here. Paul ran onto the balcony to tell them to hurry and by the time he stepped back inside the head was born. It was amazing to feel it there. Paul quickly checked to make sure the cord was not around the baby's neck, then ran to switch the stairwell light on for David and Jude.

He was back in time for the baby's leg to slip through his hand. As he tried to catch him he fell from me into a dish we had sitting there. Jude appeared at the doorway to hear me cry out 'I've dropped him' (all through the pregnancy I felt this baby would be a boy). Jude ran over and scooped our beautiful son up in her arms and gave him to me, commenting how long the cord was. Everything had happened so fast and best of all my wonderful husband had delivered our son!

After the placenta was born we hopped into the bath and David floated Daniel in the water. I was in shock and couldn't stop shaking, however the bath soon calmed me.

So our little son whom we named Daniel Wayne was eager to come into this world. He weighed 3.4kg and had dark hair, a beautiful round face and gorgeous blue eyes. We then cuddled up together for the night.

BIRTH AT HOME

Baby Cassie: born on a mountain

I've twice delivered babies for Angie, winding my way up the long, slippery road full of hairpin bends to the isolated house, perched right on top of the mountain, with views down into thousands of forest trees. It was easier the second time as I had a four-wheel drive for the journey. But the effort was worthwhile, because Angie and Ron had put so much thought and effort into preparation for the births, which is clear from Angie's own story.

She makes some excellent points about being responsible and realistic about home birth. And another thing that strikes me on reading her story is what she says about children at the birth. This confirms my own impression that children cope much better when faced with reality. It's nice to think that kids like this will grow up with the idea that birth is a normal fact of life.

Angie's Story

There is so much I could write about my first pregnancy, labour and home birth, but I have decided to concentrate on the important things I learnt from my experience.

Of course the lovely and familiar home environment, the warm bath, the daffodils and jasmin, the raging fire, the sweet smelling massage oils, the companionship and help of my birthing team, the jokes, the pain, the breathing, the waiting, the walking, the first sight of my baby, the look on my husband's face, his pride, his horror, the champagne, are all my special memories which are very valuable to me, made possible by labouring at home.

However, in retrospect, two and a half years after the event, the issues that particularly relate to home birthing, which seem important for me to convey to expectant mothers planning a home birth are as follows:

- the value of taking responsibility for my own labour;
- not being disappointed when I failed the superwoman test;
- the incredible amount of attention, love and assistance I received from my birthing team;
- the need for a good support system after the birth.

When my labour began the head of the baby hadn't dropped and it was definitely not engaged and I had had very few, if any, pre-labour contractions. Consequently my labour was quite long and slow. After fifteen hours of regular and fairly painful contractions, David (my doctor) examined me and said I was now well engaged and maybe just one centimetre dilated.

I was of course most depressed by this news as it seemed I had been having contractions for such a long time now. As my labour had started at 1.00 am I had missed a night's sleep and was beginning to feel tired. It was at this point I got a bit angry and more determined and decided to make the contractions really hurt. Six hours later my baby girl was born, so I suppose the change in my attitude and my determination hastened the whole proceedings.

I believe it was at this point that I became totally responsible for my own labour and I realised it was only me who was doing the work and feeling the pain, and that no one else could really do it for me. This became an important decision for me and a turning point in my labour from which ultimately I gained a lot of personal strength. I believe that by taking this responsibility I developed an attitude which enabled me to become a happier, dedicated and more willing mother. This of course was only the final step in a process which was started in the first days of pregnancy. I had begun conditioning myself for the arduous and demanding task of mothering by my actions of caring for my body and foetus, changing my diet, resting and restricting myself.

The decision to have a home birth was another step and the completion of a natural labour was the final one. Although this can be achieved in a hospital environment by a strong and determined woman, there is a tendency for mothers-to-be to subconsciously or sometimes quite consciously hand over the responsibility of their labour to hospital staff and doctors.

When the labour becomes a bit tough, long or painful the mother expects relief from drugs, epidurals and in extreme cases caesarian section to solve her problems. Besides the myriad of complications associated with these intervention methods on the general health of the mother and baby, they also seem to me to be a cop out.

Although it may be argued that to endure pain which can be relieved is an unnecessary suffering, I really feel the labouring toughens a personality to enable a mother to cope with the rigorous demands of a new baby. Ultimately both mother and baby will be happier. In the end the decisions made by me during my pregnancy and labour are the same ones you have to make when caring for a small baby. The baby is your total responsibility and although the father will help, in the final analysis it is really up to you.

Logically, it seems, having made these decisions during labour and pregnancy, the transition to motherhood will be easier. So in summary, I believe the value of taking responsibility for your own labour, which is easier to do in a home birth situation, allows for a great deal of personal growth and strengthening, which can only assist in the transition from a carefree single person to a selfless mother.

This brings me to the second issue I wish to discuss. Before my labour I was very optimistic about my abilities and after having taken responsibility for my labour, felt disappointed it took so long and hurt

HOME BIRTHS

so much. I anticipated (as always) that I was superwoman and I was, of course, upset when I failed to live up to this. I believe that my lack of experience played a major role in this perceived failure and had I been present at some previous births I would have been much better prepared for the whole deal.

This is another important feature of home birthing, as it allows fathers, children and friends an opportunity for close contact with the birthing process and hopefully younger girls will not be so naive and totally isolated from labour as I felt.

Also I believe there can be too much emphasis placed on painless labour by some members in home birth and natural birth circles. Encouraging a woman to take responsibility for her labour is different to giving her unrealistic expectations of how she can control her labour. Home birth attendants need to be aware of the fine line between the two.

Perhaps painless labour can be achievable by intensive preparation, meditation, and skills like that, but if this is not your style do not be conned into equating home birth with painless birth. Should you need to be transferred for a caesarian you can always take comfort from the fact that you had the opportunity to attempt a natural birth and the failure to do so is not such a big issue, as you still took responsibility for your own labour.

The feeling of dissatisfaction with my own labour only lasted a short while until I realised what I had actually achieved. I had a beautiful daughter who was well bonded with myself and her father, in a pleasant loving and caring environment. It was really a great success and the length and intensity of the labour became irrelevant.

The third point I wish to mention is the superior care and attention I received from my birth team. Present were a doctor, a midwife, a student doctor, my husband, my sister, and a friend, all of whom were there totally to attend to my needs.

The midwife stayed with me for seventeen hours while the doctor visited twice during the day and spent the last five hours of the labour and a few afterwards for the cleaning up and celebrating. It would be hard to imagine such absolute attention given to someone in hospital.

Lastly, because you will not get the care after the birth that you would get in hospital, e.g. meals, washing etc, it is necessary to have a well-organised support group to take care of the household for you. Superwoman failed again and needed, at the very least, six days bed rest. Before the birth I hadn't thought too much about what would happen immediately afterwards, but it became obvious fairly quickly that in my first week I was totally occupied with resting, recuperating and establishing breastfeeding and that all my other needs had to be met by my husband and family.

I wouldn't change my home birth experience for anything and feel very privileged to have been able to have had such a wonderful opportunity and am now looking forward to my next home birth.

A first baby for Chris: full moon rising.

Chris makes her birth at home on the farm sound so simple and smooth, which is how I remember it. She used water as a labour medium and this had a lot to do with the ease of her birth. The thing is, of course, the majority of home births are easy and quick. It makes you wonder why there's so much fuss about it.

Chris' Story

It was the first month of spring and the full moon in my belly was waiting to shed its light. My pregnancy had been joyful and healthy with daily long walks up around our country lane. In the last month I had many tightenings that were strong and regular as I walked. The baby's head had connected at thirty-two weeks, so all was satisfactory. All I had to do was wait for the birthday of my baby.

Dr David Miller is a man who exudes calmness and gentleness — all my visits were like going to see a mate with a mutual interest — we'd talk about boats and the ocean, his children or whatever current affair was buzzing through the Byron Shire. I felt a strong spirituality in this person and was honoured at having found this man to handle my home birth. I had a tangled medical history when it came to my reproductive system, leaving me with only a quarter of an ovary and the year before this pregnancy, a still birth in a hospital — I was determined to have a live healthy home birth.

On 18 September I awoke with a blood show. I rang David and he asked all the pertinent questions such as blood amount, contractions and how I was feeling. He told us to be peaceful and loving and he would arrive at lunch time. I called to my girlfriend Cass who was to be a helpful companion — my midwife and David arrived together and of course the father of the child to be, Bruce, was goggle-eyed and attentive.

David decided to rupture my waters as he was a little worried about the blood show. An uncomfortable feeling having them ruptured but not at all painful. I made everyone a cup of tea then — stage one labour began.

Cass prepared a bath which I lay in, being pampered and soothed during this stage. By the time I reached transition I was on another plane. Everyone seemed surreal — I was aware they were there but had no desire to communicate. I made signals to be taken to the bedroom that I had so lovingly prepared for this day. The contractions were strong — but I remember being told that 'contractions are like catching a wave, you swim hard to get to the crest, then you ride it down'. I found myself on all fours as I was able to rock to and fro to relax in between the body bashing. Then the urge to push — such a strong desire, but I breathed through it till David gave the okay. Minutes later it seemed I was holding on to my child — a boy, who let out one wondrous yell upon arrival then looked around passively at his new world.

All in all it took four hours to give birth. My placenta came away with the next contraction and I got up and had a shower.

My fondest memory is the new dad walking into the bathroom with his newborn and saying to him, 'This is the bathroom and there's your Mama!'

The Water Birth Alternative

It was so good getting into the bath, the sensations were so heavy that I knew it was going to be very painful — then as soon as I got in the bath it was virtually painless. Everybody stopped running around and was focusing on me. Even while most of the baby's head was out it felt really comfortable.

Nicole, mother

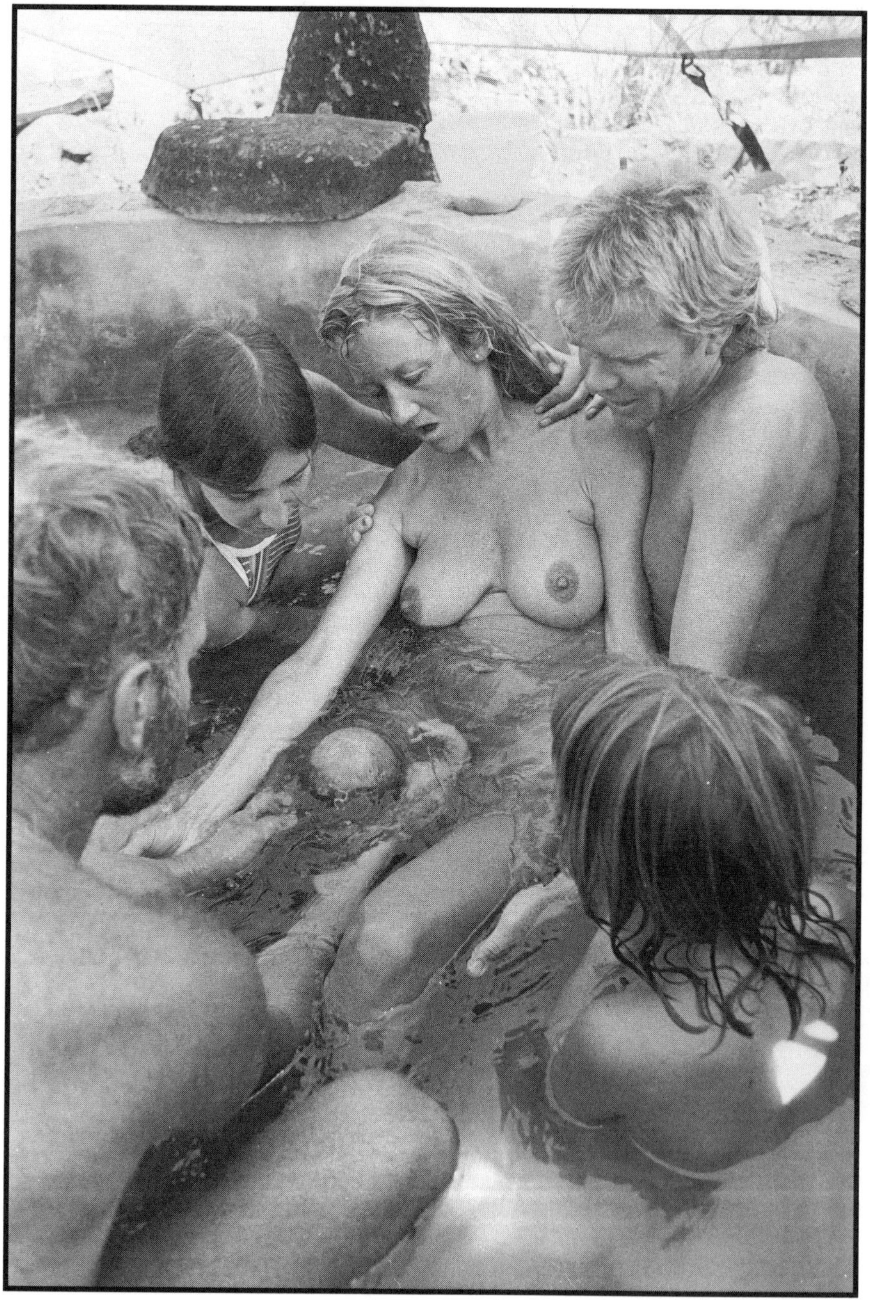

BIRTH AT HOME

THE WATER BIRTH ALTERNATIVE

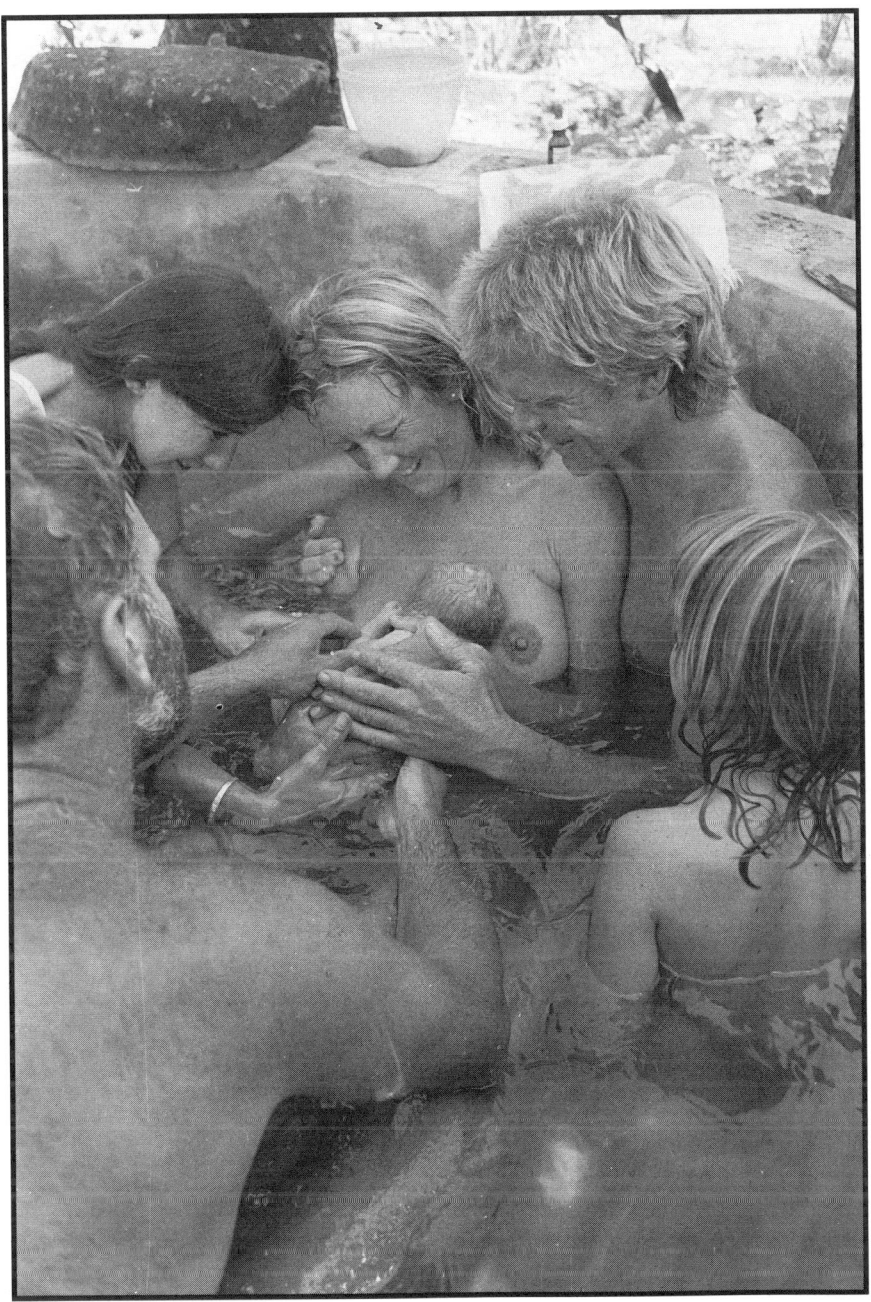

BIRTH AT HOME

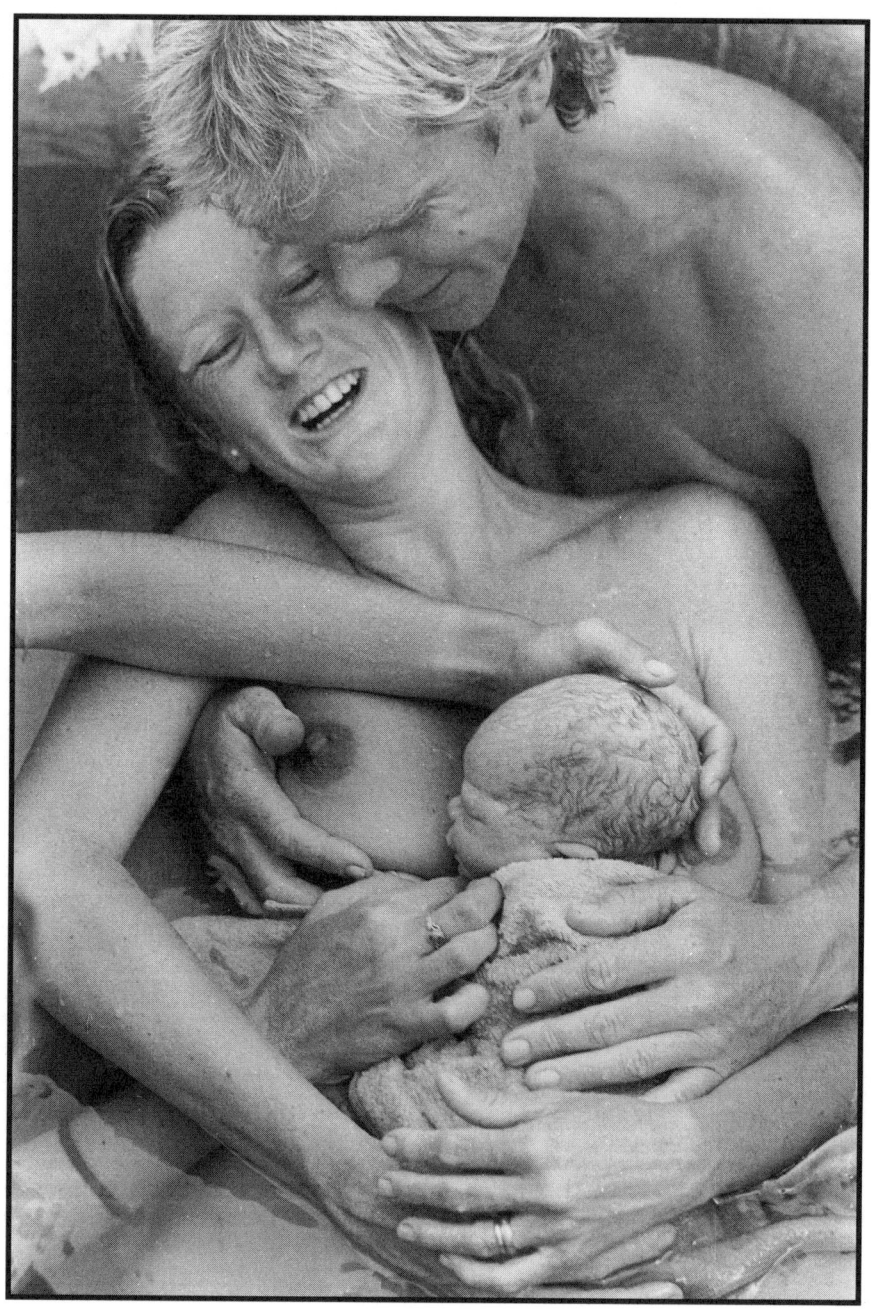

Mereki: my first water birth

In 1985, I was put to the test when Suzy and Martin approached me during an ante natal visit and told me of their plans and the wish to deliver Suzy's third baby underwater. Martin had already planned a special pool and Suzy had a good labour history.

I had recently visited the clinic of Dr Odent in France and seen video tapes of water birth in Russia under the care of Dr Tcharkovsky. I had observed that these babies seemed to survive the immersion with no apparent discomfort — but to actually supervise such a birth myself caused me some anxiety. As a doctor in a small community, my home birth activities were controversial enough. If something went wrong with this, I thought, all hell would break loose.

However, Suzy's history and the attitude of the whole family was totally supportive and I agreed to be present. As in all home birth situations, I brought along a full range of safety and resuscitation equipment and planned for all foreseeable emergencies. Two skilled assistants were present.

As part of the pre-birth visit to the home I checked out a pool in the garden, where a tarpaulin had been rigged up to keep out the sun (but not the wind, which I realised later was quite important).

The birth, which followed two weeks later, was for me an incredible experience, because it was a first and because it was so different to any other birth I'd attended. The baby was born in salty warm water, and came to the surface some seconds later. (At this early stage, of course, while the baby is briefly under the water, it is getting oxygen the way it was in the womb — the air passages are still full of liquid as they were in the womb.)

The day was windy and there I learned a practical lesson. It's not just the water temperature but the ambient air temperature that is just as important to control.

Any new baby needs to be kept warm and a wet baby, lying 'between wind and water' (sailor's talk), can rapidly lose body heat. The problem was quickly remedied in this case by covering the baby with a warm rug. Mother and baby soon moved into the house, still attached by the umbilical cord.

By the time I came to this birth I had worked through most of my doubts on a theoretical level, by watching videos and by discussions with the very experienced water birth practitioner Dr Odent in France. But in practice, on this first occasion, my own inexperience meant that I was still anxious about this new method so that, for example, I was still slightly thrown by having to rely on feel rather than on seeing the baby when it first appeared and there was that urge to get the baby more quickly out of the mother than I normally would, rather than trusting enough to let the water birth take its course.

These days, of course, I'm completely at home with this way of birth. Having this first water birth work so well gave me the confidence to continue.

Suzy's Story

Having agreed to write about our daughter's birth I am now discovering how difficult it is to capture such an event on paper. Mereki was born at 12.28 pm on Saturday 23rd, at our home, underwater, in a pool we built especially for her arrival. (The pool is an inground cement pool, the depths vary from 150mm to 100cm and it's a rounded kidney shape approximately 270 x 330cm.) The water was heated to just below body temperature by immersion heaters with our hot water supply for reserve. We used approximately 4kg of sea salt to slightly salinate it.

She was born after a two-and-a-half-hour labour, which we feel was greatly enhanced by the last half hour in the warm water. I had laboured with Martin (father) and Pam (midwife) and my two other daughters aged 6 and 3 years whilst walking about the garden until things seemed more 'serious' (we'd been having quite a giggle and getting extremely high — naturally). We decided that the baby was going to join us very shortly. We all slid into the warm pool only twenty-eight minutes before she was born. The water helped make the final and more intense stages of labour more comfortable for us both, I'm sure. The ease of movement and feeling of buoyancy were great (squatting and kneeling were easy in water).

When a baby is born into warm water it is similar to the conditions in the uterus and the baby, of course, still with the cord as it's 'life-line', does not need to breathe until it reaches air. We feel that the first breath is of the utmost importance and being born into water seems to give the child time to relax again after any 'birth trauma' before having to deal with that all important 'first breath'. Mereki did not cry or seem at all distressed as she 'surfaced'. As her cord had been around her neck loosely, but also around one shoulder, the pulse in it stopped quite soon so she was brought up sooner than we had planned. We have some beautiful photos taken by John McCormick of these special moments.

I feel it's important here to suggest that if anyone feels that underwater birthing would suit them, that a great amount of planning and learning be undertaken by the parents and birth attendants. Any fear or anxiety can be transmitted to the baby and we feel this is the greatest danger to be overcome.

Our doctor, who arrived in time, seemed impressed (this being his first completely underwater birth) with the possibilities of water providing a relaxing alternative. Many women have since experienced the soothing effect water can have on a contracting belly!

My children enjoyed the birth and 'swim' immensely, and my sixty-five-year-old mother, who has been present at both my other home births, is quite sure, to quote, 'that within ten years underwater will be an accepted way to give birth'.

We have been greatly impressed by the work done by Dr Michel Odent in France and Igor Tcharkovsky in Russia, Igor has been underwater birthing there for twenty years, and the films on his work are inspiring.

Mereki (her name is Aboriginal and means peace-maker) is one week old today and we have had her in water every day since her birth for at least half an hour. She loves water and already responds positively even just to the sound of it. She is as placid and happy as any baby I've known.

I feel well and so happy to have had such a fulfilling experience. Martin is the same. Childbirth can be a very positive and spiritually family experience, and well worth consciously working towards whilst you are pregnant and ideally even before conception.

Suzy's Mother — Betty's Story

On March 23, 1985 my twenty-eight-year-old daughter, Suzy gave birth to her third daughter, Mereki, 3.4kg, 8cm in their warm, salt water garden pool.

It was the greatest thrill of my life, to see that tiny head crowning underwater. The nasty pressures and discomfort in that final stage were taken from Suzy by the warm water. It shortened the labour and Mereki was born with ease and peace, with the loving support of Suzy's husband, Martin. I have been at all three home births and I know in my own heart that in the years to come underwater births are 'a must'. Suzy was only in the pool from 12 noon 'til 12.28 pm when her doctor and midwife Pam gave Mereki her wonderful start in life. It was their first underwater birth too, so we were all on 'cloud nine'. I thank God for the joy and happiness of this wonderful birth.

Suzy was our first woman who wanted a water birth. Her motivation convinced David to attend and see what happens. We learnt as much as we could beforehand, but there wasn't much available. Suzy had a good birthing history — easy two – three hour labours — no problems. The birth of Mereki underwater was a new beginning in birthing for our team. The ease of birth and the comfort the woman felt was obvious. We learnt the lesson of temperature control — in air and water — at this birth. The birth was outside in a spa pool and the wind was quite cool. We put our hands on the baby to keep her warm. Being born in water was just the beginning for Mereki. Water babies spend a lot of time in and around water.

PAM, MIDWIFE

Birth in the hidden valley

Expecting her first child, this young, beautiful and diminutive Sri Lankan dancer started labour three weeks early. It was midnight Sunday.

During the pregnancy she had discussed with Pam, her midwife, her strong attraction to the idea of labour in water, but because she was early nothing was prepared. There was no bath in her tiny cottage amongst the trees. What a house: unusual, very cosy, sitting on long poles and nestling in the side of a small hill, all wooded around with camphor trees. The verandah at the front of the house is high off the ground and creates the feeling of being in a tree house. The entrance at the back leads out on to a wide level pavement all made of bush rocks. Access is over a long walking bridge made of logs which crosses a little valley and connects on to this paved area.

Early on Monday morning I came with Pam to visit and assess the labour. As soon as I entered the house I saw that Jacqueline was labouring quite intensely with contractions every five minutes and getting faster and stronger.

While this was happening I happened to glance out of the window and to my surprise I saw an old cast iron bath crossing the bridge being carried by four men, one on each corner. It was obviously a very heavy and awkward burden and the men breathed a sigh of relief after they crossed and put it down onto the paved area at the end of the bridge. It was propped up with sticks and stones right there outside. A gas bottle and burner ring were produced and an old fashioned tin with 'bread' embossed on it was filled with 20 litres of water and set to heat.

After half an hour the warm deep bath was ready and 3kg of table salt were added. Sea salt is usually used but due to the premature labour we had to improvise. The table salt seemed to do just as well in preventing the 'sultana fingers' of prolonged immersion as well as acting as an antiseptic.

By now the labour was very strong. Jacqueline was well and truly ready for her bath. She was hot and perspiring and the sensations seemed to be really intense. After a contraction finished, Jacqueline was helped up by willing hands and assisted in the short walk outside to the waiting bath. She managed to get in just as the next contraction started and settled gratefully into the water which enveloped her labouring body.

I did wonder whether the training discipline of Jacqueline's ballet career might cause resistance to the necessary surrender of instinctive labour. But these concerns were unfounded as she laboured without obstruction or fear. She was supported very closely by her husband, Akram, a most sensitive man. As a couple they were well practised in yoga. The benefits of these practises were obvious in the manner of their relaxed concentration.

A strong spiritual feeling and a sense of devotion present in this couple imparted to the house, the people present, and the labour a very harmonious atmosphere. Pleasant aromatic oil burned in a dish near the fireside. Brass buddhas and devotional images were inside and out in the garden as well.

Labour proceeded smoothly through the morning hours, outside in the bath. After she had been pushing for some time it seemed there was a hold up. The baby's head would not proceed 'around the corner' of the pelvis on to the mother's perineum for crowning. We had to do something. Jacqueline was helped out of the bath onto the stone pavement. She was assisted into the supported squat position

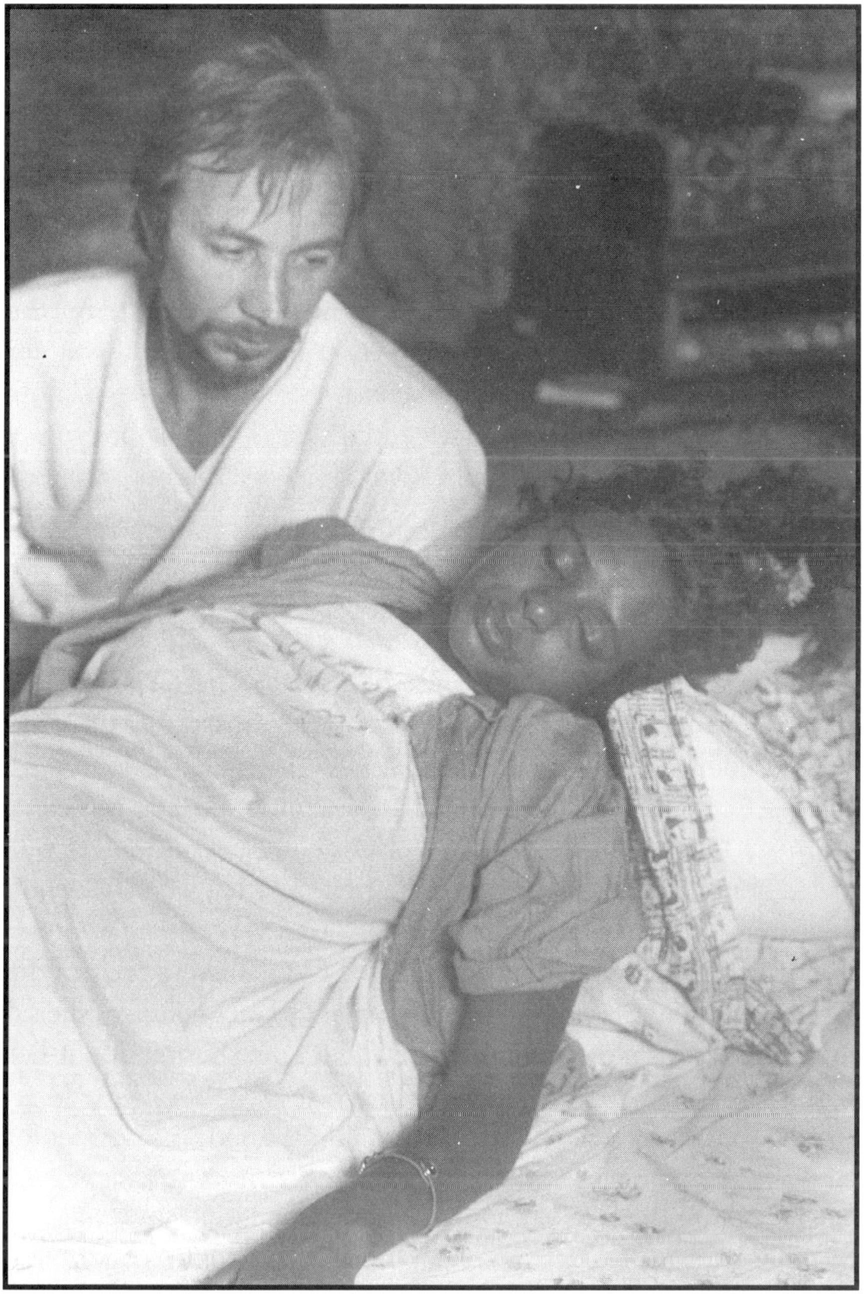

THE WATER BIRTH ALTERNATIVE

with her husband on one side and a close male friend lending his back on the other. This very powerful labour assisting position helped to overcome the problem after about eight contractions. A useful technique to help avoid the need of forceps. With progress restored, Jacqueline strongly wanted to return to the bath where she totally relaxed and delivered a 2.5kg son head first into the water.

The baby starting moving his arms and the umbilical cord was felt to be pulsing, but only slowly. So the baby was delivered out from the water up to his mother's tummy and covered with a bunny rug for warmth. He was not yet breathing. It was necessary to clear all fluid and mucous from his nose, mouth and throat. The little boy took a few shallow breaths and the pulsation in the cord became stronger. I noticed that this cord was short and care had to be taken not to stretch or tear it during the next step of transfer of mother and still attached baby into the house to a prepared warm, dry bed. At this stage the day was still and very warm — it was just after midday.

After they had settled down and while waiting for the placenta to deliver, I went outside for a breath of air and noticed that the wind had picked up all of a sudden and that low dark scuds of cloud were pushing into the clear blue sky. Half an hour later the most ferocious storm was howling and heavy rain was lashing around the now tightly closed house. Amazingly this was the first rain that we had seen in three months and was to be the breaking of a severe drought. Akram and friends prepared a luncheon feast so I cancelled the rest of the day at the office. During the afternoon I asked Jacqueline as she sat comfortably in state nursing her new son how she felt about her birth.

'The water was so wonderful,' she said. 'While I was waiting for the bath, the pains in my back were getting so intense that when I finally got into the water the relief was instant and I felt so relaxed. I don't know how I would have managed without it.'

THE WATER BIRTH ALTERNATIVE

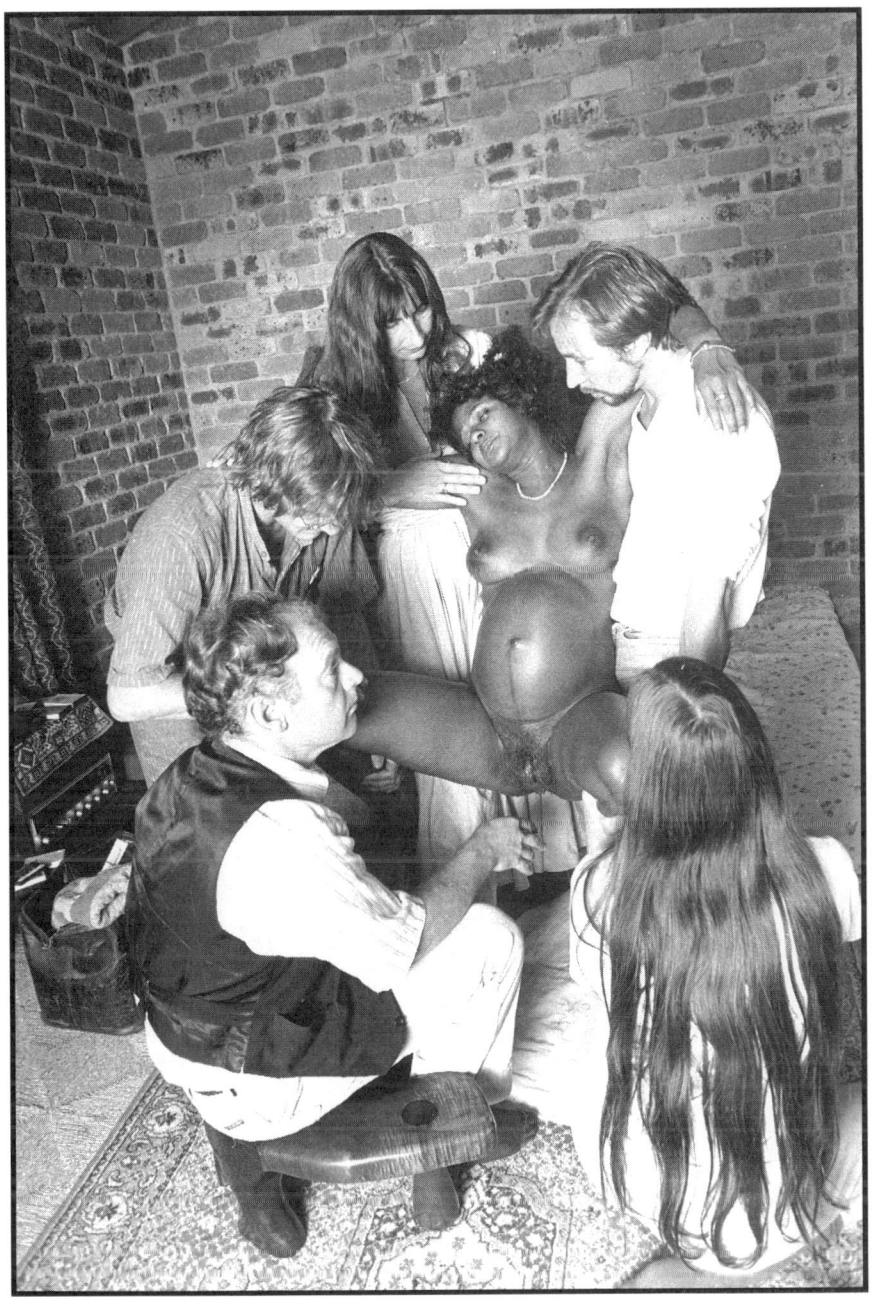

I do feel that home birthing is a much deeper and stronger commitment than most people realise, especially for midwives and supporters — it is more a commitment of the heart. So many people are very anxious to support at a birth but are quite surprised at how tired and drained they feel afterwards, especially after a long and drawn-out labour.

JUDE, MIDWIFE

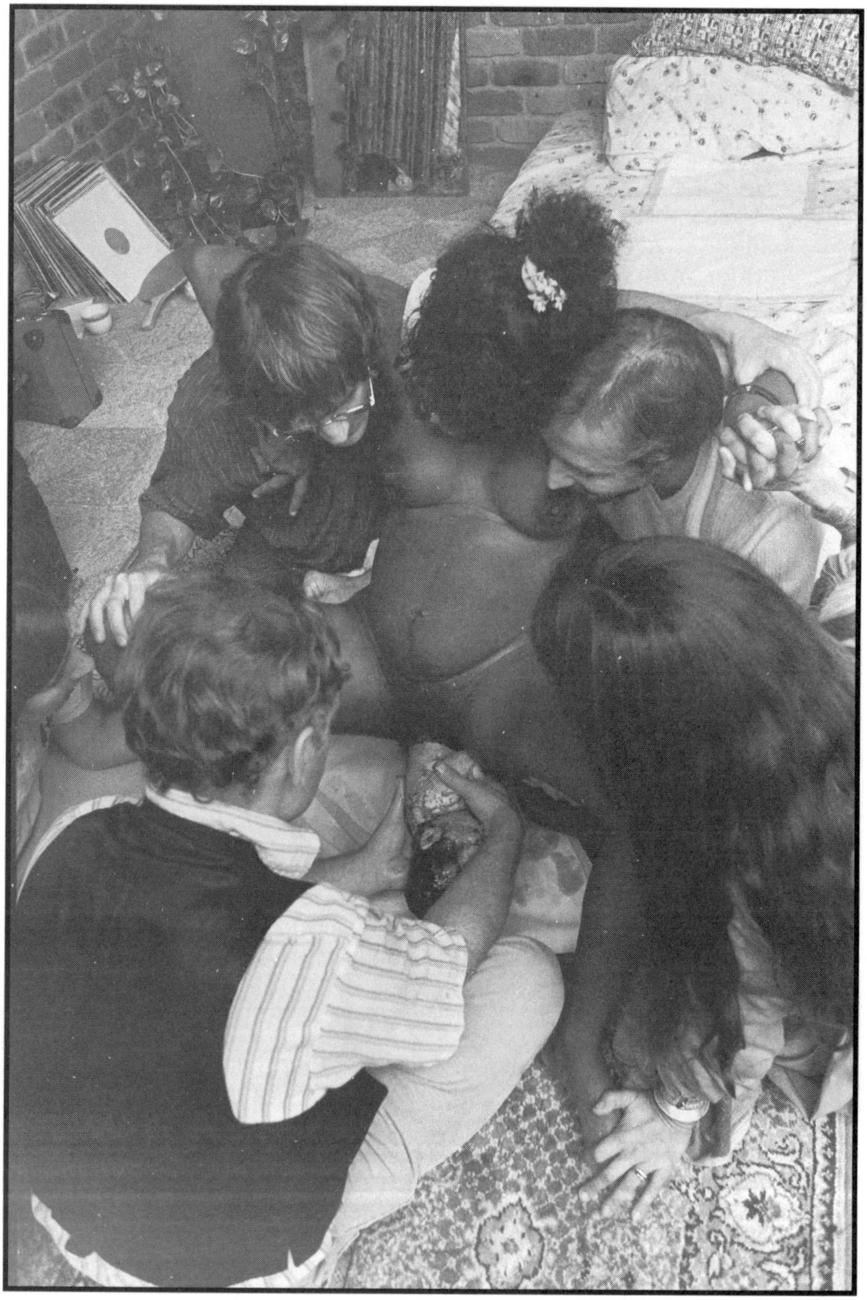

BIRTH AT HOME

Nisa: a family birth outdoors

When the time came to attend this birth, I was well used to the different ways and means of this district. In spite of the very relaxed and unusual approach to the birth, all the safety equipment was there as usual. Planning was excellent, and a bath had been set up by the family men on a specially built wooden platform in a sheltered corner of the garden, not far from the house. The temporary plumbing delivered lashings of hot water from an old but efficient chip heater.

The day was warm and still, perfect conditions for this rather large gathering of the extended family. Everybody contributed in lots of different ways. As well as Trish and her labour, there were mouths to feed and children to organise.

Too many people at a birth can sometimes be very distracting and interfere with the labouring. Most women feel the need to be very private. See how Trish finds seclusion in the midst of all these people.

Trish's Story

Nisa was born on a hot and sunny day, the last day of spring — 30 November, 1988. She is a water baby, delivered at 12.10 pm in an old cast-iron bath outside in the garden. We were extremely lucky with weather and timing — everything went so perfectly, even the fact that David, my doctor, was on a school camp the previous evening — five minutes from our farm! Pam, my attending midwife, travelled the length of two valleys (approximately 35km) to get to us.

I started labour at 10.30 pm on 29 November during an impressive electrical storm. By 1.00 am Pam had arrived and I had seen David at the camp. I had also rung my family and friends who had been invited to witness the birth. My contractions, although regular, were quite mild. After two of my sisters and their families arrived from Queensland we all went to bed to catch a few hours' rest. The contractions slowed right down and enabled light sleep. By dawn more friends had arrived and the day began with a light breakfast and walking. It was a perfect, sunny, beautiful day in the most wonderful valley nature could provide. We live on a farm with seven families, so four of us went visiting — the contractions were still mild but consistent.

By 9.00 am we returned to my home, David was there, and after an examination, determined the cervix to be 4cm dilated. I felt the need to be with Patto, my man, so we set off for another walk alone. This I found very calming and the closeness was warm, loving and exciting. We stopped at one of the houses and passed the 'progress report', then back up the hill at a leisurely pace. Contractions were becoming more intense.

By 10.30 am we were back home where there were lots more people by this stage. After another examination my cervix had dilated to 7.5cm and David advised rupturing the membranes. Pam agreed so I placed my trust in them. When this had been done I had a cold shower, then an enema, laboured with contractions for half an hour outside, then went to the toilet.

I felt very calm and relaxed — no fear and was enjoying the experience. Hiske, my girlfriend, was giving me Reiki (healing by touch) through the next series of contractions, which I found a great comfort, along with the deep breathing technique — deep breath in through the nose, down to the abdomen and expelling through the mouth, releasing pain and tension. I was still labouring outside with an audience of small children, all waiting for the big moment of the baby coming out. My two sons, Terry and Saul, were present and I felt very good about this. By 11.30 am the contractions were demanding my concentration and I needed to be with Patto. We walked to the other side of the garden together, squatting on the way during contractions. The waters were releasing and the contractions were coming 30 seconds apart and lasting for 90 seconds. Being with Patto during these long hard contractions gave me extra strength and support. I felt very close to him and could feel his loving energy. We were joined by Hiske, and another friend Vicki.

During contractions Hiske gave me Reiki and Vicki rubbed my back and I leaned on Patto. In between contractions we talked and joked. Pam and David came over and thought it a good time to get into the bath, if I wanted to.

At about 12.30 pm I got into a clean, warm, salted bath. The bath was outside in the garden with a large tarpaulin over the top to protect us from the sun.

The feeling of finally getting to the water after all these months of waiting and preparation was very rewarding. Immediately I felt relief and ease and it gave me something else to focus myself on, other than my breath. I found the most comfortable position was either squatting or kneeling forward. I had an unfortunate contraction lying back against the bath —I felt helpless and incredibly uncomfortable in this position, but fortunately that was the only contraction in that position.

I was aware of a lot of people around the bathtub, it seemed like mostly small children, but rather than bother me it made me feel more aware. All the faces I knew and loved, and also the adults who were present were dear friends and family, and their energy also gave me strength. However, I needed to be touching Patto and have him right next to me, as if we were literally experiencing all these sensations simultaneously. He was with me all the way! I felt we were one together and our friends and midwife were still rubbing my back, pouring water over me, wiping my face, and breathing with me.

I felt the endorphins release, a tingling sensation on my face and body and an airy, spacy state of mind. I knew it was close by now — the contractions were gripping and then I had the first bearing down sensation. David was there and could feel the head. The next bearing down contraction I experienced, I panted rather than pushed because of fear. I explained to David that I was too scared to push and he told me to feel for the baby's head with my hand. I did this and felt the head — the next contraction I pushed with my hand still on the head. I felt her moving down, coming towards me — I seemed to be drawing her to me as well as pushing her into my hand. I took a breath and pushed again, she didn't stop — I took another breath and gave one more almighty push and she shot out into my hand I was so amazed by this that I couldn't believe it and couldn't even open my eyes to see her for myself. I was still recovering my breath, then I could hear people telling me to 'look, open your eyes and see'. I opened my eyes to see this huge 4 kg baby floating face down in the water — all bluey/white and all there — perfect. She floated for 60 seconds like this until Pam and David helped me turn her over — she started to cry immediately, loud, strong, healthy voice — David cleared her nose and mouth and Pam put her to my breast. I felt ecstatic and Patto's face reflected my own feelings. The energy around the bath was electric.

I want to emphasise the difference between hospital and home birth and recommend a home birth most highly. Nisa is my third child and her's is by far the most satisfying, fulfilling birth. There is a stigma attached to home birth because of the old conditioning that women are afraid to trust themselves unless there is a doctor present, who half the time doesn't make it anyway. Both doctor and midwife at home were not the dominating factor and stood back for family bonding, but were there when needed.

Shirley and the seven babies: birth on a bus!

A country doctor never knows what to expect next and I was certainly taken by surprise when Ron and Shirley rolled up in their bus-home to enquire about home birth. As all their children kept pouring out the door I could only think of the woman who lived in a shoe. It turned out that this very together family had been living like this in perfect harmony for years As the family grew, the bus had to get bigger.

The birth history of any woman is most important, in order to work out the likely outcome of the one expected. Shirley's story is typical of many women actively seeking natural birth, in that she had previous awful experiences. As she became more experienced herself, her births became smoother.

Home birth for this family meant in the bus. And she wanted a water birth as well, as this bus boasted a fine bath. Sometimes I think I must have seen all the possible home birth combinations, but this one took the cake!

As Shirley describes it, the bus was parked in my yard during the waiting days, and what an asset this family proved to be as they filled in the time planting trees, fixing the water tank and mowing the lawn for me.

Here it is, a long story, one full of life and experience. We can learn a lot from women like Shirley.

Shirley's Story

I have had seven children, every birth being a different experience. At twenty years of age I gave birth to my first child. I was young, naive and unmarried. I started in labour at 7.00 am in the morning and took myself off to the hospital. At 12.00 noon that day I was taken down to the labour ward, where my legs were strapped up in stirrups. I was then encouraged to bear down and push, by a handful of nurses. I did so until 5.00 pm, when exhausted and with my face half covered with a gas mask, I was given an episiotomy and I gave birth to a 3.5kg baby boy — a nightmare birth but a beautiful baby.

My second child's birth, eight years later, was better as I was determined it would be. I went into labour sometime in the afternoon. Labour progressed slowly and by 9.00 am the next day I left for hospital. At 10.00 am I was prepared: shaven and given an enema, then taken to the labour ward. Labour by now was strong and I was ready to deliver, but the doctor had to be found on the local golf course. I was told to hang on — and try crossing my legs. At 1.00 pm the doctor arrived and told me to hold back whilst he gave me an episiotomy. Holding on was impossible, and my baby slid out with such force it nearly landed on the floor. He was a tiny 2.7kg baby boy. The doctor had said that the baby was premature and the day before had given me tablets to stop labour, which I refused to take.

For my third birth two years later, after all these problems in hospital, we considered a home birth, but were still reluctant. When labour started about 10.00 am I just continued with my chores.

By 4.00 pm labour was very strong, but I was going to spend the least time possible in a labour ward, so we stayed home. By 5.50 pm labour was very intense and we took off for hospital. We had just about reached the hospital gates when my waters broke and I caught my baby in my hands under my skirt. What an experience, but really beautiful and blissful. My 3kg baby girl was born with the cord around her neck which my husband casually removed. Everything was fine until the nurses appeared and the cord was briskly cut, and

THE WATER BIRTH ALTERNATIVE

my daughter whisked away from me. I did not see her again until breakfast next morning. I tore slightly.

Baby No. 4, two-and-a-half years on. I was being treated by a specialist as I had miscarried twelve months earlier. I had had enough of hospitals, doctors and nurses so we left town looking for a midwife for a home birth. We lived permanently in a bus by this time, and it wasn't quite suitable for a birth, so we moved into a friend's house. Labour started at lunch time and we went for a walk along the beach. Labour was well on the way so at 6.00 pm we walked back to the house. At 7.45 pm I gave birth to a 3.5kg baby girl. She also had the cord around her neck. Our hospital-conditioned midwife panicked, this being her first home birth. She cut the cord instantly, causing delay to the baby's breathing. It took a while for her breathing to stabilise — then she gave us all a smile and made the birth as blissful and calm as we had hoped.

Again I had torn with this birth, but applied the grated root of comfrey plant to the perineum. It healed with four or five days and my skin retained its elasticity.

Now I was up to my fifth birth two-and-a-half years later. This was to be my first birth in our bus which we had acquired, and had renovated enough for a home birth. Labour started at 1.00 pm and progressed like the others. As the labour wasn't intense the midwife stayed home. When she arrived at 7.15 pm she said we would have an 8 o'clock baby. At 7.45 pm my waters broke, drenching my husband and the midwife. By 7.50 pm I had delivered another baby girl, 3kg. By now I had two boys and three girls, and a happy and proud husband.

Baby No. 6 again two-and-a-half years later and another home birth. Sunday afternoon we took a long walk along the break-wall. As we made it back to the car my waters broke. We went home and labour didn't start until 2.00 am in the morning. I had an incredibly beautiful experience, feeling for the first time my baby's head connect in position for birth, and instantly the onset of labour. I lay in bed till 5.00 am then got up for a protein milkshake. Our bus was quite crowded, but we had it very organised. As well as my husband, myself, and our five children, the midwife had her two children with her. I sat on my bed until 7.00 am. We started to prepare for the birth as labour was quite strong. At 7.10 am I said I was ready.

At 7.45am I delivered another beautiful 3kg girl. The best and easiest birth of all. She also had the cord around her neck, but it was gently unwound. Everybody blissed out at the simplicity of it all, and by 8.00 am everyone had calmed down and were all eating breakfast.

For my seventh and latest baby we planned an extended holiday so decided to have this one further up north. We found a doctor who did home births and also water births. So the choice was ours.

We moved our home on wheels to the doctor's yard! On the day of the birth we drove to the beach. I felt slightly uncomfortable and was reluctant to swim. At 12.30 pm I went down for a swim. It was beautiful, comfortable and very relaxing. I stayed there in the sea for twenty minutes then we went up to the bus for lunch. As we reached it I felt labour was starting. I showered, then all of us (almost eight) drove on our bus back to the doctor's backyard. My eldest son, seventeen, was not with us for this birth.

My pains had progressed to 2-3 minutes apart. It was now 1.15 pm. By now I realised I'd seen the doctor's car back at the beach, so on our arrival we telephoned the midwife. I knew that if I stood up I would deliver. My husband started to prepare for an air birth delivery himself, as we knew nothing about water births. I asked him to run water into our bath in the bus, and prepare for a water birth also. At 2.00 pm the children were all looking concerned. I told them, 'It hurts, but it's OK.' Just then the midwife arrived and helped me into the bath. The water was about 100mm deep and we continued filling the bath until it reached my armpits. The feeling was incredible. The pains seemed to have disappeared and I felt like my labour was stopping. The midwife instructed me to push with the next contraction and I would deliver. What a contraction! I felt my tummy tighten and managed a push — the waters broke. I pushed again and delivered another beautiful baby, a 4kg girl.

I couldn't believe it! The largest baby yet and the most painless and easiest birth I had ever expected to experience. It just felt so comfortable, so right, so natural. It would have cut the pain of labour by about 80-90 per cent, and would have to be the best way for a woman to give birth. If I had realised my doctor was on the beach I could quite easily have delivered in the ocean.

The stress and anguish that I usually feel at birth — obvious in my facial expressions — were eliminated in the water and this, in turn, removed the anxiety from the faces of my husband and children. They were more relaxed which in turn relaxed me. I will be forty-one soon — twelve days after my seventh birth. Ross and I have five girls and two boys. Our eighth baby will definitely have to be an ocean birth, time and weather permitting.

Albie: the almost-finished home birth

I remember Gail's determination to have a home birth, as she and Rob, her husband, were in the throes of finishing their new house while meanwhile living with their four children in the shed.

I never had any doubts about Gail's ability to deliver her baby. As she points out, it's her fifth son. I expected her to be knowledgeable because of her work with the Nursing Mothers' Association and the help she had given many women in breastfeeding. Her awareness during the birth is reflected in her very lucid description of it.

Gail's Story

Albie is our fifth son. He is now eighteen months old. He was born at our home, underwater, in our bathtub, after a two-hour labour. In the lead-up to the birth, my husband Rob and I were confident and happy to have David and Pam deliver our baby and were ready to enjoy our first water birth.

My waters broke at 9.40 pm. Contractions started about forty-five minutes later, when Pam and David arrived. The contractions began five minutes apart. As they became stronger, we talked and I paced around, leaning on furniture when contractions happened. Pam rubbed my legs and back. As contractions became stronger, Pam asked me would I like to get into the bath — yes please! Rob filled our old claw foot bath — it seemed to take forever. As soon as I got in the bath I felt the urge to push. It was an experience that I'd never had in my four previous births. Instead of feeling uncomfortable pressure on my buttocks, legs and pelvis, I was floating and could feel my baby sliding down the birth passage. I felt that I knew where he was as he moved down. His head was born, then, after a pause, his body. His cord was around his neck and body. Dr David and Pam unravelled him, underwater, in a lovely somersault. I've seen this done before with air births and it has looked clumsy, but Albie looked so natural rolling underwater. I picked him up from the water and we put blankets around him. Those first moments of genuine bliss are just too hard to describe — every parent will know them!

After the cord stopped pulsing, Rob and the doctor helped me carry Albie out to a mattress on the floor, his cord was cut, and Rob nursed him as I delivered the placenta by myself. I thoroughly enjoyed the water birth. The water dulled the intensity of birthing. I would have another water birth.

Two Years Later
Albie is very placid, calm and easy going. He is shy, but confident with himself. He's happy, affectionate and has been a total delight. He loves to have lots of skin contact with both of us and his four older brothers, who love him heaps. They love to play with Albie and he enjoys being included in their games. He is starting to speak and he said: 'Albie! — he's a little beauty.' I think that says it all! I am so glad and grateful that I met Pam and Dr David and that they were there to help us bring Albie here for all of us to know.

Yaan: waterbirth by the ocean

Originally I had intended to be with Vicki in her house by the sea, but was away at the time of the birth, which was attended by Dr Karel, a new member of our team. I was extremely pleased to be able to share her experience of the birth through this description.

Vicki's Story

The sound of waves crashing around rocks and lapping over sands had a wonderfully calming effect on me during my labour. The medium during my contractions and for my child's entrance into the world was water and as each contraction built up, the sounds of the ocean on my birthing tape helped me stay centred and at peace while I worked with my unborn child — still snug in his watery domain.

I finished my midwifery training very sad and disillusioned. Pregnancy, birthing, the parent-child bonding and aftercare seemed to be fraught with so many unnecessary rules, regulations, irresponsible actions, and pain. I was quite determined never to fall pregnant.

Now ten years and three children later it is more than clear to me that to have the happy, healthy, marvellous experience that women are so privileged to be a part of they must take total responsibility for every aspect of it.

Obviously if complications become evident during pregnancy, specialist care is needed to work with the mother to ensure a pleasant, safe birth, but not to detract from her vital role as the nurturer of the unborn child.

I found the loving support, care and understanding from the doctors and midwives involved with my home/water birth was very reassuring. Often (seemingly) overworked and underpaid it is obviously a 'labour of love' and I feel very lucky to have had such wonderful people to support me.

From the ante natal period to the post-natal aftercare everything is geared to satisfy the mother's individual needs, and to ensure a safe, loving environment for the mother and baby, unlike the hospital birth where the norm is to satisfy the doctor's needs and the hospital routine.

As well as the doctor and midwife, my mother, two sons, and the baby's father were present during the birth, and in their own special way all contributed to the beautiful, peaceful atmosphere that filled the house. My mother had never seen a child being born and to have the opportunity for us to share this special time is something we will always treasure. In a lot of ways it has created a beautiful new bond between us.

My contractions progressed rapidly with the rise and fall of the ocean sounds — my backache was soothed under the warm stream of water coming from the shower, and from there it seemed a natural progression to step into a bath to complete the final stages of my labour.

Yaan came from water and was born into water and it felt so safe — so right. His strong little legs were frog kicking as he made his way, aided by the midwife, to my abdomen. As his head emerged from the water he opened his eyes and greeted us with such a calm, blissful look that it filled me with joy. He stayed in my arms and suckled while his body still floated in the familiar watery environment. Yaan spent the next seven hours either quietly sleeping or observing his surroundings before he uttered a sound — a gentle cry which was quickly silenced with a feed.

My mother's initial reaction to her grandchild being born underwater was one of horror, but as her understanding and confidence grew towards Yaan's birth she proved to be an invaluable support for me. She did a wonderful job photographing Yaan's birth through her tears of joy, and together with Jude, my wonderful midwife, Paul — Yaan's very special daddy — and his two big brothers, our lovely child was born non-violently and unintrusively into a place where he was obviously at peace.

Isaan-Julian: a supportive second birth

Birth can be an intensely spiritual experience. For me, the elation and charge that I feel coming away from a successful birth can be so energising as to overcome fatigue from lack of sleep. So many babies are born just before or around sunrise. Driving home through the country on a misty morning after such a birth is one of life's delicate moments.

The feeling at Susannah's birth was very strong. A single mother, she was ably supported by good friends. In preparation for the birth, a bath was somehow carried into her upstairs flat and placed on the enclosed verandah. As part of the pre-birth home visit, I had the supports checked under the verandah before the bath was filled. A full bath is very heavy and the spectre of bathwater, baby and all crashing through the floor was too mind-boggling to contemplate.

Susannah mentions how she touches the baby's head while it is still in the birth canal. She is employing a very effective bio-feedback technique to allow her to know exactly what she and the baby are doing and give her more control over her labour.

The description of her first baby's, Martino, birth is interesting, because although the labour seemed quick and straightforward, she did not have the right support to allay her fears. During the birth of Julian, the constant support from her friends gave her all the confidence she needed.

BIRTH AT HOME

Susannah's Story

Baby, I waited so long for you, then you came so quickly that I could hardly believe holding you. When I woke up having a couple of contractions, as so many nights before, I just turned around and kept on sleeping. Forty minutes later I was wide awake. Eleven o'clock. I timed myself for about fifty minutes before actually believing that I had gone into labour. It was time to phone my friends and get Jude and David to come.

It is midnight, starlit sky. My rushes are getting stronger and more frequent when David checks me. I am already 5cm dilated. Everybody is getting things ready, it's a wonderful atmosphere in my living room, everything seems perfect.

I feel the baby pushing down strongly and Jude makes me get into the hot bath. Water over my tummy — it feels so good. It pushes down so strong, it hurts. Jude reminds me my baby is coming! I don't even have to push, I am all breathing. I'm opening up more and more, and then I feel the head pushing through. David makes me touch it — my baby. The shoulders push through and there is his little body swimming out of the security of mine into the water. So free! I am craving for him. I hold his little body. I feel so much love. This is Julian! He is so peaceful, so relaxed. Slowly he starts breathing. No cry. No shock. What a gentle birth. It is 2.10 am, 13 October, 1988.

My mind travels back to nine years ago — Martino's birth. Extraordinary, simple. A little cottage on a south Italian island. Candlelight, an Italian midwife, old fashioned, insecure. No centre. I can't keep my breathing together. Four hours' labour — an easy birth, but I get frightened in the second stage. The midwife is no support. My baby slides out. I am lying on my back. I am exhausted. Don't cut the cord — she does it anyway. She doesn't give him to me. We are crying for each other while she cleans us. Finally I hold him. I love him so much. He is dressed. I have to undress him to feel his little body. It is 1.05 am, 3 July, 1979.

THE WATER BIRTH ALTERNATIVE

Alana: a midwife delivers her daughter

I first met Andrea at the local hospital professionally, where she was an experienced and sensitive midwife. So when she came to have her own baby I was honoured by her request to be present. As it turned out, her husband Geoff, her sister Deena and her close midwife friend Sharon Currey supported Andrea so well that I had no great role, other than as emergency backup.

Andrea delivered her new daughter with her own hands, so expertly. It was most satisfying for me to watch a woman take such total control of her labour.

P.S. Andrea has since delivered a son, once again catching him herself, with the same loving support, in the same beautiful timber family home. And Sharon is now a member of our birth team as a result of these encounters.

Andrea's Story

Alana is our second daughter. Our first daughter Mia was born three years earlier in hospital, and although a very positive hospital birth we had decided that this time we would have a home birth where we could just be ourselves.

We were very excited to find that I was pregnant, particularly because I had had a miscarriage three months before, which I found quite devastating at the time — it really felt that I'd lost a baby and needed to work through the whole grieving process. This I was able to do with support from Geoff, my sister and close friends.

During the first few weeks of pregnancy I did feel nauseated at times and tired, but once I reached fourteen weeks this passed and I began to enjoy my pregnancy. One problem that I had to deal with during pregnancy was a slight anaemia and vitamin B12 deficiency which was rectified with oral chelated iron and an injection of vitamin B12.

Another problem was varicose veins and a vulval varicosity which were quite tender at times. Oral vitamin E helped as did wearing masseur sandles and yoga. I always put my legs up when sitting and witchhazel helped reduce the swelling and tenderness.

During my pregnancy I began to think about the possibility of delivering the baby myself and to giving birth in water, which sounded a natural medium for the baby to be born into. She had spent the last nine months in a watery environment. We have a big cast-iron bath which seemed the perfect place to deliver. I have been trained as a midwife and I think this helped me to feel confident about helping our baby to be born. I was remaining open minded about all this as I didn't know how I'd feel when the time came.

Alana was eight days overdue and two days prior to her birth I was really feeling I'd like her to be born soon. I felt anxious to see her and be with her in her new world, but always aware that she'd know when the time was right.

The morning had been spent down at the beach swimming and playing on the sand. Late that afternoon I started to get backache every fifteen minutes. My sister, Deena, arrived to stay the night and it was with great excitement that I went to bed at 9.30 pm still having slight intermittent contractions.

I was not to get any sleep though. I was in bed until midnight and then started getting up and going back to bed again — I had diarrhoea and by 1.00 am needed to be up — the contractions were

5 minutes apart and I needed to rub my back. Deena got up with me and took over the back rubbing — it was nice to have her with me, there is a special closeness between us. Deena really tuned into my needs — applying just the right amount of pressure with her back rubbing.

Geoff stayed in bed trying to get a couple more hours sleep, but I think he was just too excited to sleep. At 3.00 am Deena rang Sharon (a close friend and midwife) and Geoff took over the back massage. I felt I'd like to be examined just to know how things were progressing. Sharon arrived and examined me — I was 3cm dilated — it was 4.45 am.

I felt pretty much in tune with my baby, but a few negative thoughts crept in such as 'Gee I don't want to do this again'. I dealt with these thoughts and let them flow in and out with my breath. I found the most comfortable position leaning over the kitchen bench and squatting down slightly during the contraction. The waves of contractions were pretty intense and felt mainly in my back. I was using sounds during the contractions — firstly ah, then why, then wide. I was sending this energy to my cervix, visualising it widening and also sending energy out through the top of my head.

I tried using hot towels but didn't really get much relief from them so concentrated on my sounds and back massage, which was great — Geoff was fantastic and seemed much more in tune with this labour and my needs.

I hopped into a very full hot bath and it was amazing the relief it brought. I was kneeling and leaning over two pillows at the end of the bath so my whole abdomen was completely submerged, which took a lot of the sensation of the contraction away from that area.

The back massage combined with the pouring of water over my lower back really relieved the back pain. I felt so much more in tune with the whole birthing process in the bath.

Sharon had rung David at 6.00 am and he and Pam arrived at 7.30 am. I was examined — 6cm dilated. It was a nice feeling to have them there, somehow the birth seemed closer. Pam helped me centre my thoughts and energy by holding my arm when I nearly lost control a couple of times.

I started to get the bearing down urges and at about 8.45 am. I was fully dilated and ready to deliver. I felt clear and positive about delivering the baby myself so I half knelt and half squatted in the bath with towels under my knees and feet for comfort.

The bearing down urge was amazing and I gave a couple of good pushes, feeling Alana's head descend fairly quickly. I then breathed, grunted and made animalistic noises rather than push and her head came out slowly — I still felt that burning stretching feeling, but maybe not as intense or for as long as with Mia's birth.

Once Alana's head was born her body followed quickly — David said she somersaulted. I then picked her up and lay her on my tummy with her head down. She was very alert at birth, requiring only slight suctioning.

Wow! what a buzz — a little sister for Mia. I then got out of the bath to deliver the placenta after about 45 minutes.

I started walking around in the garden and then half squatting, half kneeling delivered the placenta.

Mia was really great during the whole labour and birth. She woke herself at about 3.00 am. I felt my thoughts actually wake her as just a minute before she woke I said to myself 'I'm pleased Mia is getting some more sleep'. She wanted to come downstairs and she cruised for a while and then fell to sleep for a short time upon the bean bag. She really handled things well and whilst I was in the bath she handed me the washer and then wiped my face with it. For one moment she looked as though she was about to cry so I asked Deena to take her outside for a while and she played happily with Damien (Sharon's son).

I was then ready to deliver so Deena and Mia obtained a great view poking their heads through the bathroom window.

As soon as Alana was born Mia came inside again and she was happy and certainly not distressed by the event at all.

I'm so pleased she was such a part of it all. I know it has made the bond between Mia and Alana even closer. I could see the love on Mia's face as she held Alana and Alana seemed so peaceful and relaxed in Mia's arms.

I am now pregnant once more and looking forward to the birth of our third child. I have felt in my heart that there was a third child for us to share our lives with.

Since having such a wonderful birth with Alana I can see no other way than to have another home birth and to have the baby in water if it again feels right.

Pam's Benjamin: the team reverses roles

I know Pam very well because she has worked closely with me as birth attendant at more than a hundred births. So when she asked me to deliver her baby, I felt as though I was attending one of my family and was quite nervous about whether my performance would be up to scratch.

Something I didn't realise until labour started was that Pam wanted me as the midwife. How I had to work! Following her around, supporting and reassuring her, just as she had done for all those women.

The strong feeling for water, so apparent in her story, may well have been the result of having been with so many women who were helped in labour and birth by this element. I understand Pam's sentiments.

I have grown so used to the labour option of water now that not to have water available for a woman would seem to be denying her a basic right. Water is not for everyone — but for the woman who feels it may help her relax, like Pam, it is a great ally in labour.

Pam's Story

I chose to have a water birth after working as a birth assistant for five years, attending home and hospital births — air and underwater. The moment any labouring woman hopped into the bath, a feeling of relief came and labour was easier — just as strong but easier for the labouring woman to integrate her breathing and control with the contractions. So when it came time to birth my first child I felt confident that the water would be the place to labour and birth in. My waters broke in the early hours of the morning and I waited until my contractions were moderate and regular before entering the bath.

My husband, doctor and friends assisted me with massage in the water and kept the bath at an optimum temperature. I hopped in and out several times — I liked the change of atmosphere and also to be able to work and squat and stretch. Each time I hopped back into the bath I would feel a sense of ease and gain my composure to continue my hard work. As second stage approached the water gave me security during the intense period of transition. I had plenty of support from the bath sides and my attendants could easily aid me. Birthing underwater was controlled and progressed with ease. I found any position of squatting sideways in the bath gave me ample room. The actual birthing of the head and body was helped by the warm salty water — my tissues stretched easily and my baby was born without stress. When the body was out my newborn stretched and then made frog-like movements towards my leg, and then I lifted him out of the water onto my chest and tummy with his head in a downwards position so fluids could drain from the mouth and nostrils.

My baby was very alert and peaceful. He looked around constantly and started breathing with small breaths simultaneously. We covered him with warm bunny rugs and I moved out of the bath to a prepared bed, and we cut the cord when it had finished pulsating. The placenta followed soon after. I continued putting my baby, Benjamin, in the water as part of his daily routine.

Benjamin is now eight months old. I found the birth to be one which has given Benjamin a warm relaxing start to life. His disposition reflects this. He has been a happy, calm baby and has a love of water. Bath time tends to be a time of learning new movements, a time to relax back into the element so familiar. Water relaxes Benjamin, similar to us having a bath to melt the worries of the day.

His motor skills are more advanced in water than air. He often discovers new movements in the water. In the early weeks of waterplay/swimming, Benjamin would completely relax into his bath and sometimes even fall asleep! It was so much like home for him as a newborn. Water on his face is no problem. Benjamin can go underwater without fear and he knows how to 'hold his breath'. Having had Benjamin in water it is easy to use water as relaxation during times of discomfort. (I put Benjamin in water on day 2 when he was uncomfortable with a bit of meconium — I also use it as a comforter when he's teething.) He is so involved with the water. Anything to do with water attracts him, from swimming, to the kitchen tap, to raindrops. It is a real delight to watch Benjamin grow loving water.

I feel that his development is normal and it is too early to say if he's an Olympic swimmer or such — it wouldn't surprise me as Benjamin's physical development is highlighted by being 'educated' in water.

Difficult Situations

Sometimes things happen
that are out of our control and we
have to accept that and help in whatever way
we can, remaining positive and supportive.
We act as guides and helpers to the family
to give them the best possible natural birth
— be it at home or in hospital.

Pam, midwife

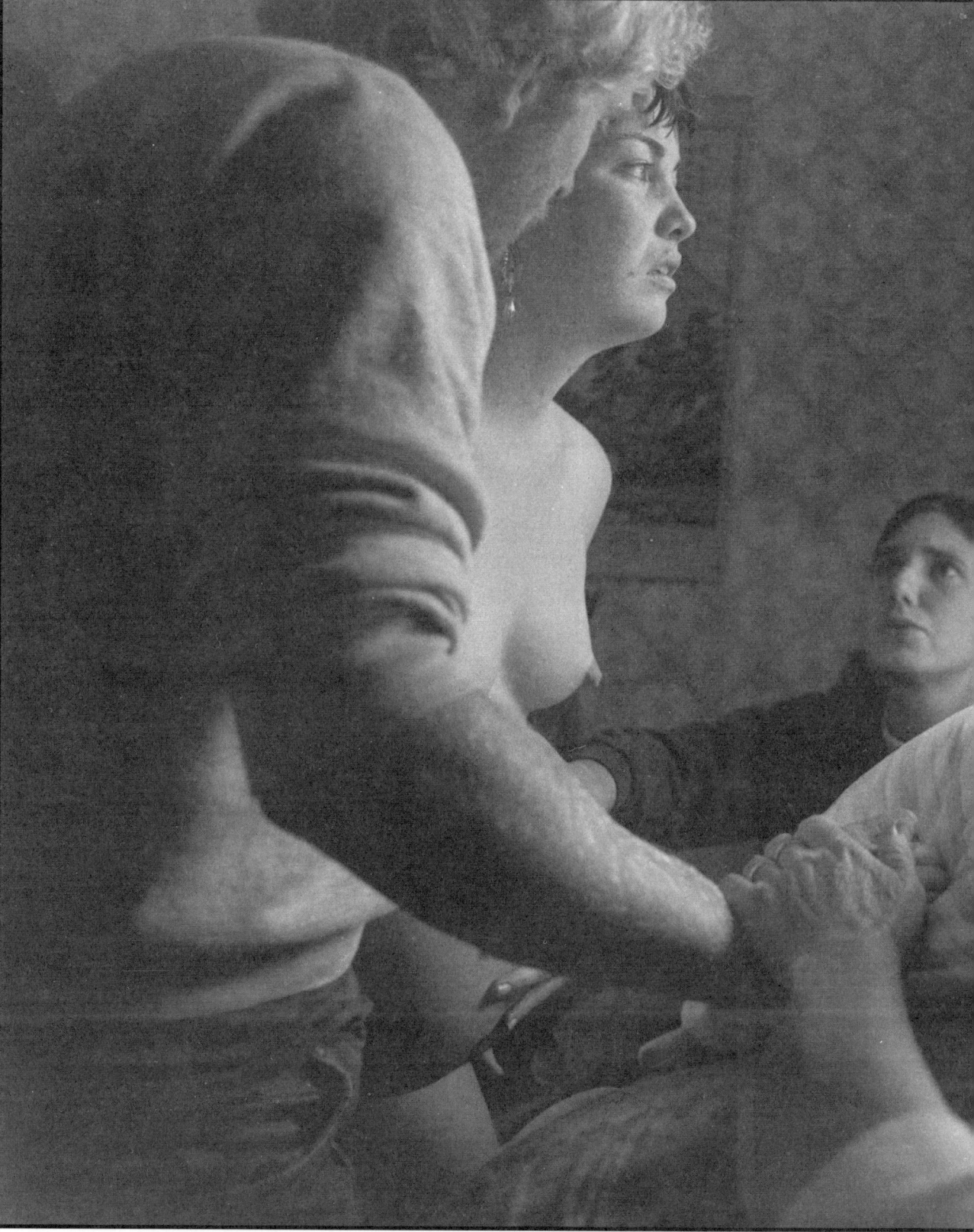

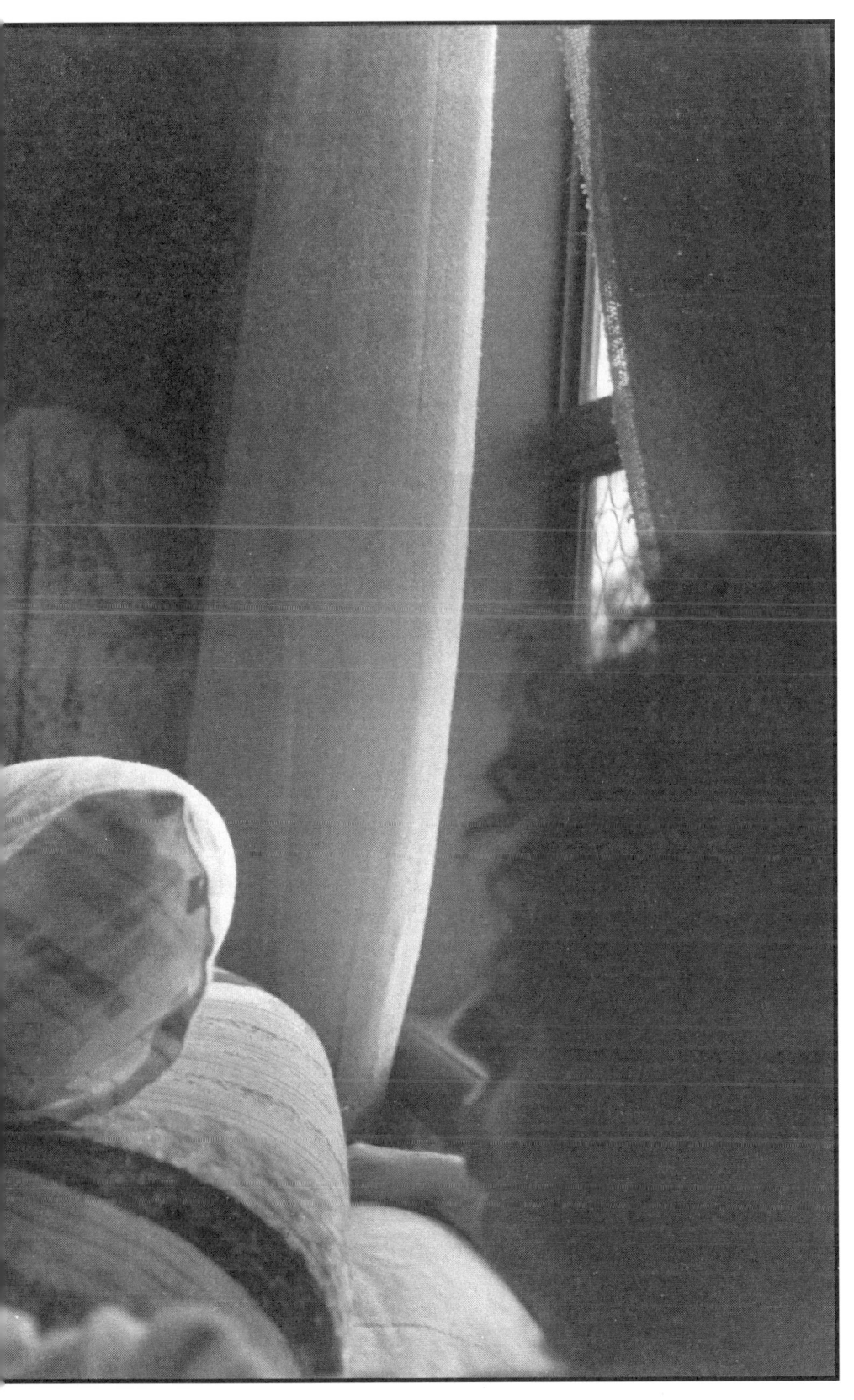

> *Fear seems to be one of the biggest problems and prevents women surrendering to labour, especially after a traumatic experience with a previous birth. I wanted to help women dispel that fear.*
>
> JUDE, MIDWIFE

BIRTH AT HOME

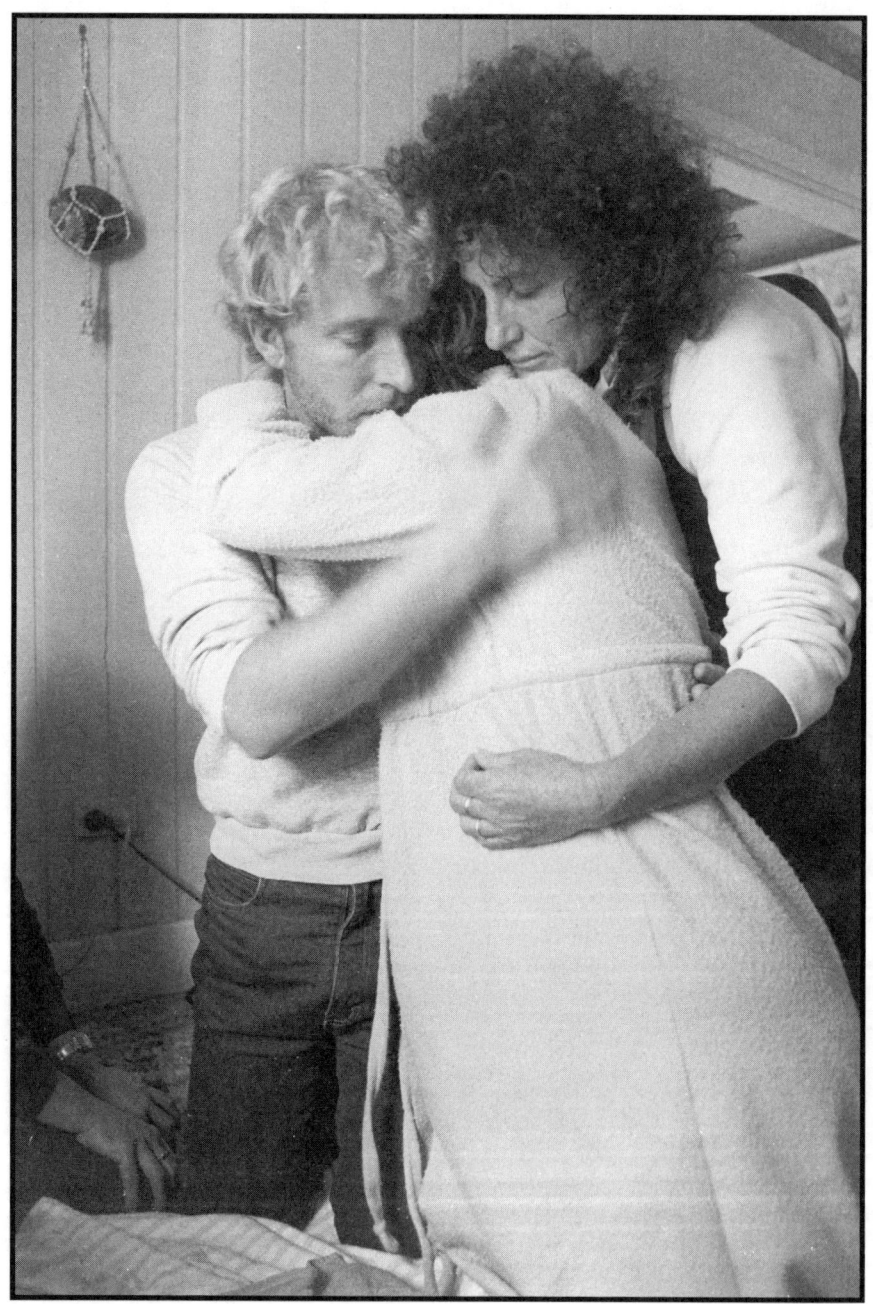

DIFFICULT SITUATIONS

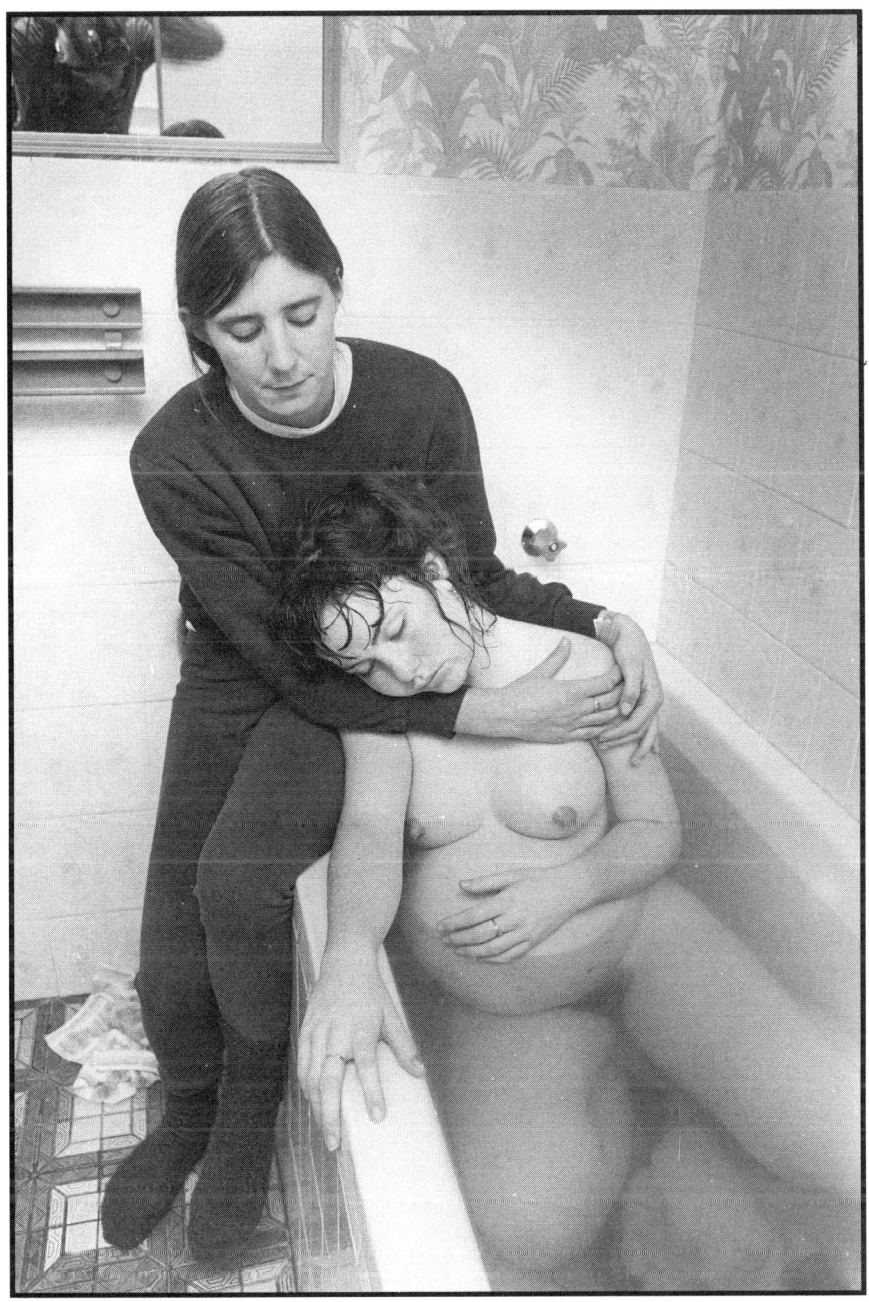

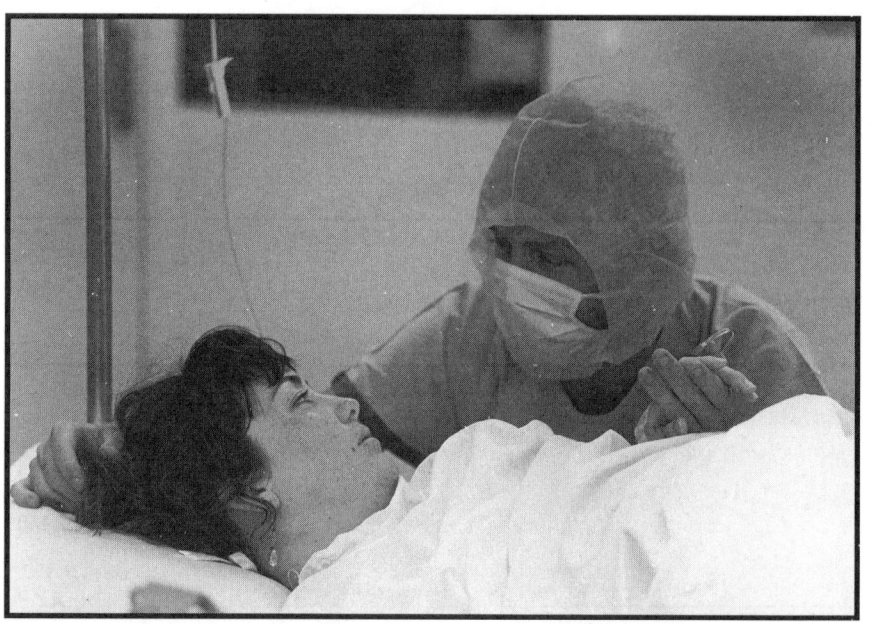

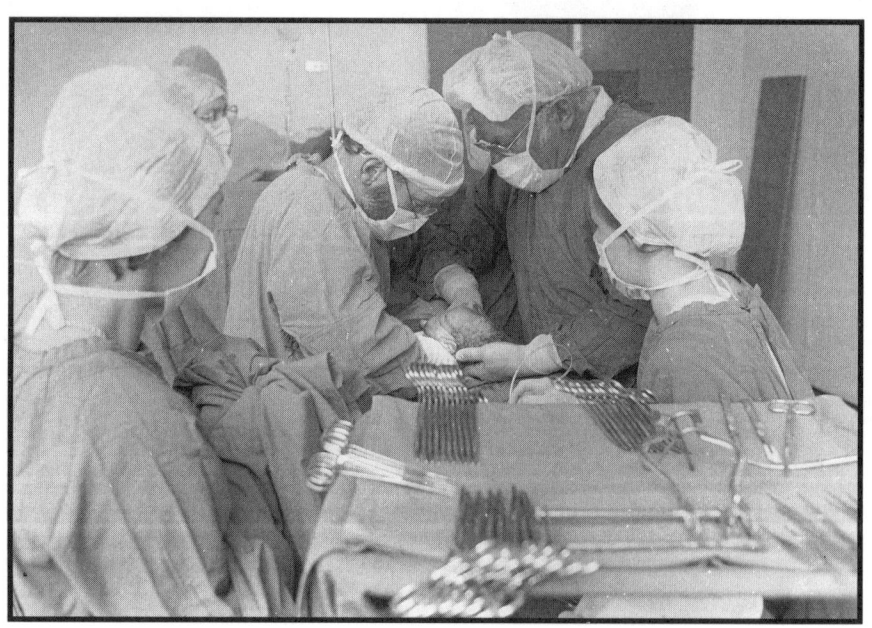

DIFFICULT SITUATIONS

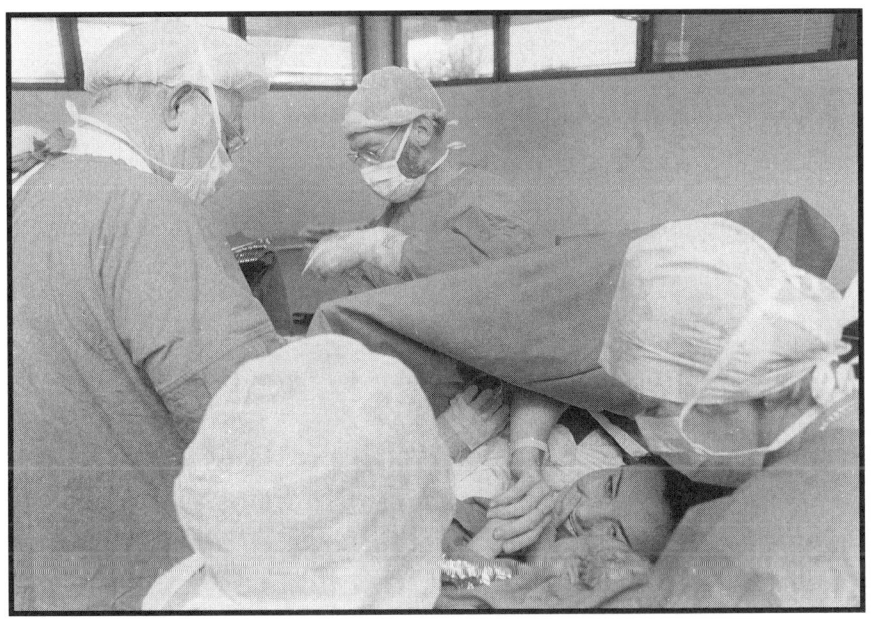

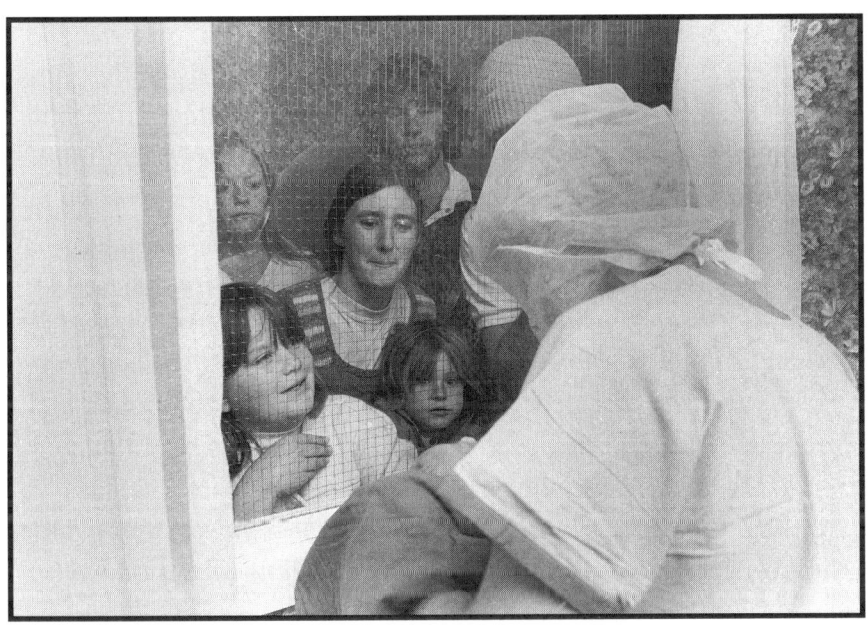

Jenny: breech at home

I have no doubt that anyone reading this will think how dangerous it must be to have a breech birth at home. Of course there are many situations where I would strongly advise against home birth — and there are occasions when I have had to tell a woman that her wish for a home birth is just not practical or safe for the occasion.

I suspected that Jenny's baby might be born breech (bottom first) when it didn't turn a few days before labour. It's not uncommon for the baby to turn head first at the last minute. Before labour there is no way of knowing whether the baby is going to turn to the more desirable head first position.

Jenny had such a good birth history, and the baby was presenting so favourably when labour started as breech, that it seemed safe to see how she progressed. As well, she lived very close to the hospital. As it turned out her labour was smooth and progressive and the baby delivered easily — every case should be judged on its own merits.

By adopting a squatting position for the delivery, Jenny had a much better labour than if she had been lying on her back, the more traditional position for 'at risk' labour.

The benefits of home birth in relaxation and freedom, which make people opt for this choice, also help to make difficult situations like this one easier.

DIFFICULT SITUATIONS

Jenny's Story

A breech birth at home! You must be mad? Didn't you make it to the hospital? How could you take such a risk?

These were a few of the comments made when told of our exhilarating (to say the least) home birth. The answers of course were No! No! and No! It was no more of a risk having the baby at home than having the baby in hospital, considering I had no complications.

As the due date was approaching fast and the baby had not turned, any apprehension we had about having a home birth were waived after speaking with David. He explained that he would do nothing different should we be at home or in the hospital, and that he always has the necessary equipment wherever he may be. The decision had to be ours and that he would gladly support either decision.

When my waters broke and the contractions started I had no thought whatsoever of running around packing bags, sending kids off, cleaning up the house, etc. etc. It was total concentration on just being me and the baby. To allow this baby to come into this world in its own time, in its own way, and in its new home with his family.

Jude (midwife) and Sue (support person) worked extremely well together, setting things up and keeping me relaxed. The pushing finally started and out popped his bottom first, and everyone yelled 'A boy!!' (an advantage of a breech is that you know the gender first off). Then David helped to pull down one leg and then the other. I must admit that I was in excruciating pain by this time and knowing that the head was yet to come I said to my husband, Bob, as my fingers dug deeper into his shoulders, 'I don't wish to do this any more!'

I then visualised myself being rushed off to hospital with my entourage of Jude, Sue, Rania (our eight year old), David, Bob and myself with half a baby hanging out. Not a pretty sight.

'Help stand her up and she'll be able to push down easier,' I heard someone say. It sounded better than off to hospital, so up I staggered with the help of Jude and Sue. With a couple more almighty pushes out popped this gorgeous baby full of bliss and joy. I found out later that David helped guide the baby down by gripping the mouth with his finger, which prevented the head from locking into any difficult position.

The baby did not breathe straight away. Bob and I thought it was an eternity — it was about a minute. With the efficiency that you expect from doctors and midwives, the oxygen tank was connected and the baby was breathing within seconds.

It was as David had said. We had all the necessary equipment, we just had to feel right about doing it. I am forever grateful to David, Jude and Sue for their support.

DIFFICULT SITUATIONS

Off to hospital

Did Marg really need a hospital birth? After all, she had not laboured for very long at home and did deliver quite easily in the end.

Marg is a good example of every case being different and the sum total of the problems meant to me that hospital was a more suitable venue. Personal problems, difficulties with her father, no male mate, a broken window letting in cold air, the need for pain relief — these were all factors and, of course, no real after care could be guaranteed.

As it turned out the hospital birth went very smoothly and Marg had a good rest afterwards. Today Marg is well, happy and settled, living 'happily ever after' with Joe.

Marg's Story

I was pregnant with my second child and I was alone. My first child was born by caesarian section after twenty-eight hours of labour, and it had taken me the best part of two years to really recover from this experience. Another caesarian and I really didn't know how, or if, I would cope at all.

My reaction was to stay away from doctors altogether. I figured they would carry me into a hospital anyway, so they weren't going to get me anywhere near one until the birth. Finally, when I was twenty weeks pregnant, after much coaxing from friends, I went along to someone who they told me was a very good birthing doctor.

Well, I guess he must have been curious as to why I hadn't showed up before that time. As I could have told him, the baby and I were both quite well, except that the baby was so big that he thought I may have twins. (I was absolutely sure about my dates, in fact there were only two opportunities for me to conceive in a period of four months.) Great! Twins would really put the lid on it. So I went for a scan, and saw what appeared to me to be a fairly healthy bouncing baby. I had refused a scan for my first child on the grounds that it was unnecessary.

David came to understand more of my emotional needs as the weeks went by. I was seriously considering adoption and I had found some very suitable would-be parents, and we were looking at legalities. When the time came to go and see the solicitor I decided that I couldn't give the baby up without regretting it for a long time.

By now I was nearly seven months pregnant. I had just moved into a house in town and I was finally getting organised. But I was very tired and always feeling the need for the support that was never there — from a man, I mean. The women around me were wonderful and that continued for a month after the birth. By far the most difficult thing for me during the whole pregnancy was trying to maintain emotional independence. No one to hold, no one to bounce your neuroses off, that sort of thing. It makes all the difference in the world to be loved by someone, and much more than that — you have a child in your womb with just the same needs.

During pregnancy I started pre-natal yoga classes, Iengar style, which I loved. These classes included some fairly strenuous exercises which were a welcome relief after being told so often during my first pregnancy of all the things I couldn't do in yoga. Doing exercise in that pregnancy didn't seem to do me a lot of good anyway. I always prefer to be doing something.

Dr David was also doing his bit with support. We had talked about my first labour at some length, and together we were preparing a sort of plan of management. He felt the yoga was important, which I was very happy to work at. I had organised a dependable friend to be with me in labour and I was arranging a sterile pack of necessary bits and pieces for a home birth. I also booked into one of the local hospitals (Byron Bay) as a possible emergency patient. By this time I was at last beginning to feel a bit more emotionally stable, or content.

The preparation of body and mind for transfer to hospital, even in the most adverse conditions, is one I will always remember. Through all this my daughter, Monika, who was all of two years old when I became pregnant, had to try and live on. She started preschool for two days a week when she was two-and-a-half, which she loved. As luck would have it, she and the preschool teacher really loved each other, and for Monika this helped to make up for what I could not give her at that time.

All my energies were needed for preparing for the imminent arrival. I didn't have the tender loving patience that I should have had for her, especially at that time. I did try to make her aware of what it would be like with a baby brother or sister, and she did enjoy moving into town. She also made some good friends at preschool which helped too, but what can really make up for being pushed aside by your mother? What could I have done? I don't know, except that I was already beyond any limits that I would have set for myself.

The onset of labour was very simple. I remember it was a very cold night — the first that winter, and for the first time I realised that one of the windows in the lounge room was missing, and there was a gale blowing through it. Monika and I were finishing our sweets when my waters broke, like a small flood. I rang David, and then my father who was to take care of Monika. I also rang my friend Ria, who went with another friend to collect some blood which had been crossmatched (a necessary protocol for the trial of labour, in case of a caesarian).

Meanwhile David had examined me and confirmed the start of labour. He ordered a hospital birth, since the head wasn't properly engaged. The local acupuncturist gave me a treatment to try to get energy moving down my body and to bring the labour on, and to make it shorter. It felt wonderful to be so well looked after. After the treatment the doctor took me to the hospital, where the nurses let me into the labour ward, which I remember as being very cold.

Shortly after, Ria and Lynda arrived with the blood from Lismore (a one hour drive each way) but unfortunately the hospital would only let one of them into the labour ward. So I never got to see Lynda.

David went home to get a few hours' sleep. Labour progressed for a few hours, but I started to get the urge to push before I was fully dilated. This was exactly what had happened in Monika's labour. The two night nurses sprang into action. They suggested some pethidine, which I had refused during my first labour. Since I knew the consequences of continuing in that direction, I agreed that it was worth a try. They rang David and he agreed to a small dose. Well, it made it easier to resist the urge to push. For the next hour I had a nurse one side and Ria on the other, both yelling at me not to push, but to breathe through as each contraction came on. It was wonderful.

Towards the end of the hour David came, looking a little bleary-eyed from interrupted sleep. It seemed to me that he was only there for a few minutes before he told me that I was fully dilated and could start to push.

It took me another hour of huffing and puffing to get the baby out, but that was sheer pleasure since I knew that the hardest part was over. In fact I was surprised how hard I had to push, but as usual it was much easier for me to do it than not to do it. As the baby's head came out David told me to stop pushing, which I did, and with the next contraction my baby was out!

David placed him straight on my stomach (the lights had been dimmed a couple of minutes beforehand), and he put a heater over him, in that position. They left us for some time like that, I think until the blood stopped flowing through the umbilical cord. I had not torn or been cut (I remember being greased and massaged at one stage).

Someone asked me what I would call the baby. I really hadn't thought about it previously since I had decided the first name that came into my head at the time would probably be the one. 'Well,' I said, 'I think I'll call him David.' My grandfather was called David. And David he is.

I remember them asking me to sit up to encourage the placenta to fall out. I think I said, 'I don't feel like doing a bloody thing.' Anyway, finally they got me standing up and the placenta obligingly plopped out. Soon afterwards I was feeding a washed David in the nursery talking to Faye, the night nurse, about adoption, but I realised that she had never been able to bear children of her own.

The next morning I discovered that it had snowed on Mt Nardi during the night, an extremely rare occurrence. The night will certainly be remembered by me as a very rare experience shared with some truly wonderful people.

Postscript. During the first year of David's life things were quite difficult. He didn't sleep for more than four or five hours at a time, and Monika went through some difficult times. She was always very loving towards David, however. Then our luck changed and we got ourselves into a happy family situation, and moved out of town with Joe. Monika, David and I are all thriving, happy and healthy. Such a change I wouldn't have believed possible.

Kristie: exhaustion after childbirth

Kristie's story, highlighting the problems which can develop after even the most perfect birth, is an important one to tell. As she points out, both pregnancy and labour went like a dream. Also for the first couple of days afterwards everything seemed to be progressing normally. So I was caught off-guard by her distress call.

In the early days of the birth team, we soon learned that problems following the birth were much more frequent than difficulties encountered at the labour and birth itself. To prevent such common problems as maternal exhaustion, feeding problems, cracked nipples, piles and crying babies, we developed a routine of monitoring the post natal situation most carefully. So what went wrong?

My failure to diagnose the extent of her exhaustion quickly enough perhaps came from being somewhat complacent, given Kristie's competent and assured handling of the situation to that point. Having been reminded of the possibility of a stressful post-birth situation such as she so feelingly describes, I learned to take much greater care in a number of ways — for example, in the monitoring of visitors. It seems that for the first couple of days, as Kristie says, the woman can be on a high, and this is often a good time for friends and relatives to make short visits. It is not a good idea for lots of people to stay in the house. Essential folk only, please. Well-meaning people sitting around enjoying themselves can be quite a hindrance.

Here are some tips:

Have some domestic help for at least one week so that the new mother has only to rest in bed and bond with her baby.

At the first indication that visitors are causing exhaustion, be ruthless. As Kristie suggests, a 'No Visitors' sign will not offend. Quite a few people have followed this advice.

The third day is often the most critical. On this day the woman needs to be very quiet to allow the milk to come. Distractions and obligations can delay or hinder this process.

Do not take the baby out to the shops, or anywhere else. This lesson was taught to us by a Muslim family, who followed their teaching for the mother and baby not to go out 'for forty days and forty nights'. The peaceful babies that resulted were rather convincing of this wisdom.

Use the support available in the community. In particular, feeding problems can be shared with a member of the Nursing Mothers' Association, which has a vast knowledge on the subject and can offer helpful practical tips.

Keep in touch with your doctor or midwife and alert them if you're not sure about anything.

Remember birth is a family affair. All the family is involved. Be watchful for the feelings of the other little ones, who may feel displaced by the newcomer. It's their baby too, although they may not always be as gentle as you would like. By avoiding sibling rivalry early in the piece, the family will more easily adjust to its new member.

Kristie's Story

It seems to me everything during pregnancy is designed to prepare one for the actual labour itself, with very little information to prepare oneself for the first initial week(s) with a new baby, especially a first baby.

My pregnancy was a breeze, the only discomfort was two weeks of morning sickness. I felt great for the most part, and my pregnancy ended with a trouble-free three-and-a-half-hour labour, from go to whoa. The last ten minutes of labour and the actual delivery of my baby girl, Courtney Patricia, took place in my bathtub at home. I can't describe the soothing feeling of comfort and relaxation that enabled me to centre back in on myself as the baby emerged through my birth canal.

For three days following Courtney's birth I was on what can only be described as a high. My child was beautiful and perfect, a joy. My goal of keeping 'control' of my birthing situation had been achieved. I felt a great sense of accomplishment: my first child, born at home in an ideally planned birth with no intervention.

And then I crashed back down to earth. My exhaustion snowballed from an incredible high to several days running on adrenalin, followed by two nights of absolutely no sleep for either my husband or myself.

This period was interlaced with arguments between my husband and myself amidst the screams of our discontented newborn baby. We had someone come to the house to do the washing and housework, which is essential with a home birth. But during the first six days after the birth we had an endless number of friends and well-wishers visiting our home. Top that off with in-laws arriving the day after the birth, followed by other in-laws from overseas arriving one week later and staying for a fortnight. It was all too much, and I finally peaked out: physically, mentally and emotionally drained. Add to that the fact that my hormones were still in a state of frenzy. I felt like I had entered a living nightmare. When I reflect back on the whole 'scene' now, as I write this, I honestly don't know how my husband and I survived those first awful weeks. My body and my milk shut down entirely. Exhaustion was the culprit, and I had no one to blame but myself!

DIFFICULT SITUATIONS

The most excruciating traumas I experienced as a result of my exhaustion centred on breastfeeding problems. I never ever considered or thought of possible problems with breastfeeding during the pregnancy. All of my consciousness and preparation focused on the pregnancy and actual delivery: pure diet, homoeopathics, pre-natal yoga, home birth support group, a total dedication to success with a home birth. I never questioned my ability to breastfeed my child. Unfortunately for me, I never educated myself about my body's post-pregnancy processes and the effects of hormones on my system. For example, adrenalin knocks milk-producing hormones on the head, and the stress and anxiety I was feeling produced adrenalin.

I thought breastfeeding as natural a human process as breathing. When reading through books to prepare for childbirth, most contained two chapters on feeding. breastfeeding and bottlefeeding. I thumbed past those thinking, 'I'm breastfeeding, no problem' . It's the same as someone skipping the section on caesarian section and having to have a caesarian. These things just don't seem to enter one's mind when blissed out on being pregnant. The experience was a mind blower. Nobody told me breastfeeding is an 'art' of sorts, and I wasn't aware of the wonderful Nursing Mothers' Association until problems arose. And when they did all hell seemed to break loose.

Totally exhausted, emotionally strained after arguments with my husband, sleepless nights and the incredibly draining screams of my hungry baby put me over the edge. I wasn't sleeping, wasn't eating, and wasn't enjoying motherhood one bit by the end of the first week. Courtney was not getting enough to keep her quiet and contented, hence her screams added to an already tense environment. I was exhausted, yet so on edge that I was unable to sleep and relax. The more uptight and tired I got, the more my milk wouldn't let down. The fact that it wouldn't come in led to a very frustrated infant. It was like I was on a merry go round and couldn't get off. I was drinking herb teas (fennel, borage, chamomile and mint), taking homoeopathics, and eating a 'milk-inducing' (supposedly) diet of oatmeal and stout. For various reasons which I won't elaborate on now, my baby went on a bottle at six days of age and settled down.

Yet I never stopped feeling I had to prove my tits to the world. After eighteen hours of bottlefeeding, Courtney and I went through the emotionally devastating dilemma of her rejecting my breast. The bottle had milk in it, and my boobs didn't, so why suck on an empty boob when a bottle was so readily available.

At six weeks after birth, I entered hospital for ten days to attempt to relactate. I ate, rested, pumped, pumped and pumped, expressed, expressed and expressed (my boobs have never had so much action in their life!). Unfortunately it was 'too little, too late', but the break away from my home environment gave me the space to reflect on the time following the birth of my baby. In six weeks it felt like it was the first time I could be alone and get acquainted with my baby.

It's easy to look back in hindsight and play the 'if I knew then what I know now' game. But in life, experience is the best teacher. I can only share with you, the reader, what I have learned through personal experience and, hopefully, help you prevent unnecessary exhaustion and emotional upheaval. My advice: follow your intuition. Others may know more about babies in general, but you know best about your baby. About three days after the birth, I intuitively wanted to pack Courtney off and head somewhere where we would be totally alone. The warning signs were there but I wasn't able to read them at the time. I lost confidence in my mothering abilities, making the mistake of thinking everyone knew more about my baby than me.

Limit your visitors to none or the absolute bare mimimum, which may very well be easier said than done. Dr David counselled me on this, but I was too caught up on my emotional and hormonal rollercoaster to heed his wisdom until it was past the point of no return, well en route to exhaustion. After I have my next baby my husband and I will hang a 'No Visitors' sign on our front door. I don't care if the Queen of England drops in bearing flowers and congratulations, no visitors.

Make sure your partner is educated and understands what his role

DIFFICULT SITUATIONS

will be, and how important his total emotional support is through the crucial early stages following birth. Both partners must be educated about the intricate chemistry affecting emotions, physical and mental well-being and proper establishment of lactation. Relax together and take the time to get acquainted with this exquisite new soul, your baby.

The labour isn't the end, it's the beginning. Once the baby is born nothing else matters for the first few weeks. Go easy on yourself and enjoy every moment of this tiny being, because they grow all too quickly.

BIRTH AT HOME

Margaret: loss of a daughter

I really admire Margaret's courage in the way she so honestly recalls this most tragic loss of her unborn daughter. Her first baby, a boy, was delivered successfully at home eighteen months earlier, and this pregnancy was progressing normally until the movement stopped, as she describes.

Booked for a home birth, Margaret decided to go through labour in the hospital, where she was assisted by Beth, a midwife who had undergone a similar tragedy herself, and who helped her to hold her little dead baby. Even afterwards, no cause was found for the death.

Her story is included in this collection of mostly very happy stories, because the stark reality of the death of a baby sometimes has to be faced. Hopefully Margaret's deeply felt account may help some woman who also has suffered such an inexplicable loss — to see that she is not alone.

Margaret has since delivered her second son and is now pregnant again.

Margaret's Story

What I'm about to tell you took place almost five years ago now. I remember it as though it were yesterday. It was my second preg-

DIFFICULT SITUATIONS

nancy; my first being a healthy baby boy. This one was a girl, that much I knew — I was a bit more emotional than with the first.

What really puzzled me was the absence of the usual dreams I would have of myself and my new baby. Call it premonition if you like, but I didn't see me with a baby girl.

This baby had spent most of her gestational period in any position but the right one and the only discomfort I had was heartburn and a few cramps at the end of a busy day of running after my eighteen-month-old 'flying fox'. Sometime during the thirty-eighth week she clawed her way around my uterus and planted herself firmly into the 'engaged position', to await her imminent arrival. A few days later she floated upwards, knocking against the inside of me, no more real kicks, just slight bumps, which could've been confused with live movement, but nothing definite. At this point I felt the loss; knew something was missing. She was gone and at the same time she was still there. I hoped I was wrong, but I wasn't. I knew and began to quietly grieve and disbelieve, knowing that if she were dead there was nothing anyone could do to bring my baby out alive.

A further nine days passed of living in an unsure hell. My body had been contracting occasionally for four days so I was more than ready to have this baby dead or alive. On arrival at hospital it was confirmed, no foetal heartbeat, which was no big news for me.

The birth itself was quite easy, not like pushing a live baby; there was no resistance — no help.

Immediately afterwards I felt the same elation as anyone who's just given birth, the only difference was the dead baby at the end of the table, and everyone in the room was crying. I held my baby and felt her lifeless body and realised there was not much point in hanging on any longer. If I hadn't held her I don't think I would've ever believed she was not born alive. At this point I still couldn't cry. I'd been crying for the past week and saw this as the end and I was glad it was over. I was mistaken, the first stage was over, what lay ahead was much worse. I wished I could've kept her just the way she was, but that's illegal. So, born on Monday, burnt on the Wednesday.

Then they gave her back in a little plastic box, where I kept her for a year before I could let her go.

There was also the question of autopsy, which to me seemed abhorrent at the time, to cut up what I'd just spent nine months creating, even though it may have given me a legitimate reason why this happened, but it wouldn't have changed a thing.

So the grieving process began with a crater-like space in my guts that could not be filled. No baby, an abundance of milk; it's hard to describe the infinite emptiness I felt. The shame and sense of failure and responsibility I felt when people asked whether it was a boy or a girl, and I said a dead one. So from being ashamed, I blamed and was blamed. Then I resented life itself for letting this happen to me; there had to be a reason.

That reason I found within myself. I now feel I was chosen to learn the deepest lesson, that life and death and everything in between is so precious. Most precious of all is that my daughter never died, she resides in my heart and I'll always remember her.

DIFFICULT SITUATIONS

Flood rescue baby: Tina's story

In the heaviest rain since 1892, the Brunswick River in northern New South Wales received an overwhelming and relentless 700mm during the first two weeks of April 1988. During this time many of the tiny townships in the area were cut off from each other and residents in the hills were unable to move out of their houses. Families were separated for days as children were unable to get home from school. Sick and injured people were marooned at home, sometimes without the telephone and rescue helicopters were kept very busy evacuating patients, where possible, and dropping help and supplies to others.

Easter Monday
It had poured all night, golf balls of rain drumming on the tin roof of the old surgery house, so loud and constant — almost unbearable — that I could not hear the radio reports on river levels. By now it had rained every day for weeks; the river outside was already lapping its banks before the night's deluge.

A look through the window at the gloomy grey morning showed the broken banks, the flooded park, and the brown floodwaters lapping the surgery garden, rocking flowers in their beds. Like many others, I was cut off from my family in the hills. The phone rang and interrupted my contemplation.

Tina was in labour. What a day to pick, and the place: home was in the Main Arm Valley — a wild place in a flood, as I was to discover. Knowing that I would not get through in my car, I called Colin, the Main Arm fire chief, who promised to come and get me in his four-wheel drive fire truck. He never arrived as his truck became caught between creeks on the way out.

This was becoming a disturbing business. The house was in an isolated position and the roads were cut off by the rain and the high tide backing up the river. Colin had contacted the local State Emergency Service by his mobile car radio, which sent down a man to tell me the news and suggested that a helicopter was the only way in and out at the moment.

Never having been in a helicopter I was somewhat dubious about this rather extreme measure, but there seemed to be no choice. So with my bags of equipment, the S.E.S. man ferried me to the showground for take-off. There was a delay, as the helicopter pilot had been diverted to the rescue of a crashed hang-glider. However, he arrived soon enough. Dressed in Air Sea Rescue orange overalls, he jumped out and ran across.

'Do you know the area at all?' he asked. I was able to reassure him that I knew it well. There was little time to consider my fear of the rotors falling off the machine as I was quickly strapped in and we were aloft, following the course of the flooded Main Arm road.

A journey which usually takes half an hour in a good car on a good day took only five minutes, and suddenly we were landing in a paddock only ten minutes' walk from the house. The pilot skilfully avoided some trees and stated 'We're solid', but the ground was very 'boggy' and he kept his motor running. Gratefully stepping out onto a somewhat slushy terra firma, I was relieved to escape from that rotor.

A fair walk, but with willing hands to carry the gear I received a warm welcome in the already familiar house. Tina, her mother and husband were relieved to see help arrive. Jude, the midwife, arrived later by walking in. As the day progressed, Tina laboured strongly and looked set to have the baby soon, so I decided to stay rather than face the risk and discomfort of walking out and maybe having a 'heli-baby'. In hindsight this would have been the better option by far.

As the day progressed the rain eased and the roads were apparently improving. The S.E.S. were on standby for evacuations by road. At about 9.00 pm that night, it became apparent that labour had taken a turn for the worse and had stopped progressing. In the interests of the mother and baby, there seemed no choice but to move out into the night, a task no one relished. It was pouring again.

Tina was having contractions. She was strong and brave throughout the whole ordeal which was now developing.

We had to walk down the hill from the house to Colin's waiting Land Rover fire truck. Tina and her mother squeezed into the front cabin with Colin, while her husband, some friends and I went on the back for a wet and freezing ride through numerous flooded causeways.

The river had dropped significantly which was just as well. Soon we arrived at the arranged place for transfer to the large six-wheeler truck, which was waiting on the other side of Wheatley's Crossing, recognised as the most difficult part of the road. There it was waiting, as arranged, glistening red in the rain, its welcoming search light reflecting across the raging Main Arm Creek through the slanting rain.

With a confident roar, the huge beast plunged into the torrent, raising a great bow wave, in order to cross and collect our precious cargo. Then it became stuck and stuck fast on a pile of flood gravel deposited in the middle of the crossing. Here was the first sign of a hitch in a smooth, if uncomfortable, evacuation.

Busy hands shovelled away the gravel in the floodlit rain, and Colin's Land Rover was hitched up to help tow out the huge truck, which was down to the axle in gravel. Tina, her mother and Jude left the Land Rover and had to continue the labour on the side of the road in the pouring rain while this operation went on.

'This is a nightmare isn't it? It's not really happening?' Tina asked hopefully between contractions.

Meanwhile, the big truck was turned around and lined up ready for the crossing back to safety. Tina and her mother entered the apparent safety of the cramped cabin and the men jumped on the back. The stream was too strong to cross on foot. The truck entered the flooded crossing and halfway across — disaster! It suddenly fell off the eroded upstream edge of the crossing, invisible underwater.

The water was suddenly racing across the deck, like a ship going down. The truck was leaning at an alarming angle unable to go forward or back, water raging right around the vehicle. For a moment everyone was stunned by this development.

We could not easily remove the passengers because there was nowhere to go, going back or forward led into the stream..

Still the labour went on.

One man who jumped overboard was nearly swept downstream by the dark muddy current. Quickly a human chain was formed. Tina's husband, Viggo, suggested running out the fire house as a lifeline and this was done quickly and efficiently by the S.E.S. team. Voice communication was almost impossible due to the roar of the passing water. Tina dismounted and entered the water. Willing hands ferried her through the chest high water to the other side.

We left the truck and started walking, stopping for contractions, while water raced knee deep down the road we were following. We came to the next and last major crossing where another Land Rover waited. Again another fire hose was run out and brought to the other side by a human chain, but there was no securing point for it.

'Who's strong enough to hold this end?' asked the S.E.S. chief, Frank. As I have a solid stocky body, I volunteered as anchor man. Experience gained from many tug-of-war games at the local pre-school and my time as a sailor now became very useful.

This creek was deeper than the last and again Tina and all her helpers plunged into the dark rushing water. It was quite a job for me to stay upright at my post with the fire hose end coiled round my body, but I knew that I must not fail or everyone would be down the creek — without a paddle.

At last we all managed to scramble ashore like shipwrecked sailors, as the welcoming ambulance beacon hove into view, giving us the reassurance that the dangerous crossing was finished, thus avoiding the Leboyer birth which I feared was imminent. Terry the ambulance officer was very comforting as we soon drenched his tidy, dry ambulance with mud and water.

On arrival at the local hospital everyone was quite shocked and, of course, wet and shivering. Surgeon's outfits were handed out all round. Then I found to my dismay that essential theatre staff were flooded in their homes and that the usual road to Lismore, the nearest Base hospital, was cut by floodwater.

I called in another doctor to help and he set up an epidural to relieve Tina's distress, in preparation for further evacuation. An alternative route to Lismore was worked out, a journey of 150km or one-and-a-half hours. All the way, the baby's heart stayed strong and Tina was comfortable, until near the end of the ride.

On arrival, a caesarian section operation was quickly organised and Tina delivered a beautiful baby daughter called Hannah.

Postscript. Two years later, I saw Tina at a gathering at which she told me of an argument she had with a friend who had declared, 'How you are born doesn't make any difference.'

'In my heart I know what she told me was wrong because Hannah has been so upset. She's starting to settle down now though, but I know that her labour ordeal and then having to be ripped out in a caesarian has made her early years very unsettled. As well, you mightn't believe this but, she just doesn't like going anywhere near the creek. I know she would be different if she'd been born the way I wanted, like all my friend's babies who are so peaceful and happy.'

BIRTH AT HOME

Tina's Story

Labour began gently enough — this is OK I thought — aha! It continued on through the night getting stronger with the rain pounding overhead non-stop. My mother came about 4.00 am to help me on my way. We planned a home birth, preferably in the bath.

The rain kept coming but I was becoming increasingly oblivious to this. By morning, the valley we live in was flooded out and a friend and midwife arrived from further up the road which relieved my worries a little. Later my doctor was flown in by helicopter and another midwife joined us, having forded the creeks.

Meanwhile the labour was getting stronger — didn't know it would be like this — racking your whole body. 'Good contractions' they call it. Hmm! Laboured on through the day — rain continued — but all seemed fine. By late afternoon it looked like Hannah and I were in some trouble — Viggo, my husband, and all around were starting to look concerned I noticed between contractions. Hmm. Hospital everyone agreed — too dark for the helicopter to land now...

Friends — a shot of pethidine — a snort of brandy — a quick pack — out into the stormy night. Thinking, 'Oh, no, this is not really happening,' but with an inner calmness a labouring woman seems to have, we went on.

My memories are of: gumboots and rain, four-wheel drives and rain, and, of course, contractions every few minutes; fire trucks, broken roads, waiting and rain; premonition of trusting my own feet. I had fears at one stage during the creek crossings — the water was waist high and running very fast — as the fire truck jerked off the side of the bridge and water swirled everywhere. I thought 'I'm not going to have this longed for baby — and I'm not going to get through to the other side — at this stage I was feeling very distressed — tired — and tired of my contractions — and I felt like crying — but there was so much commotion and things to get on with that it passed and my sense of humour returned. I couldn't crack up when all around were doing their very best — the men were in the water with a fire hose. Jude, the midwife, and my mother were holding me and on it went ... one fire truck driving across a causeway misjudged and got stuck ... of inching our way across three causeways ... of thinking how good everyone was ... and when I get to the other side the pain will go ... of my doctor standing all in yellow with a fire hose around his waist as we all inched through another creek.

And bliss ... in a dry ambulance ... more bliss at the local hospital after an epidural relieved the pain of twenty hours of labour, a few more hours — in Lismore hospital — Hannah was born by caesarian — fit and healthy — as Viggo held my hand. Thank you everyone for helping us through the unexpected.

BIRTH AT HOME

Comparative Home Birth Statistics of Two Areas in Australia

	Byron Shire, NSW 1983-1988	Bunbury Region, WA* 1983-1986
Total planned home births	142	165
Primipara (first baby)	45%	31%
Actual home births	133	130
Hospital		
Transfers for complication	9	26
Spontaneous hospital delivery	2	12
Caesarian	2	5
Newborn		
Resuscitation required	3	1
Neonatal mortality	0	1 (congenital abnormality)

* From a study by Dr Keith Howe

Byron Shire 1985

Total births	180
Planned home births	48
Actual home births	44 (24% of total births in shire at home)

Australia wide 1985

Total births	242,900
Planned home birth	1,135
Actual home birth	1,055 (0.4% of total births in Australia at home)

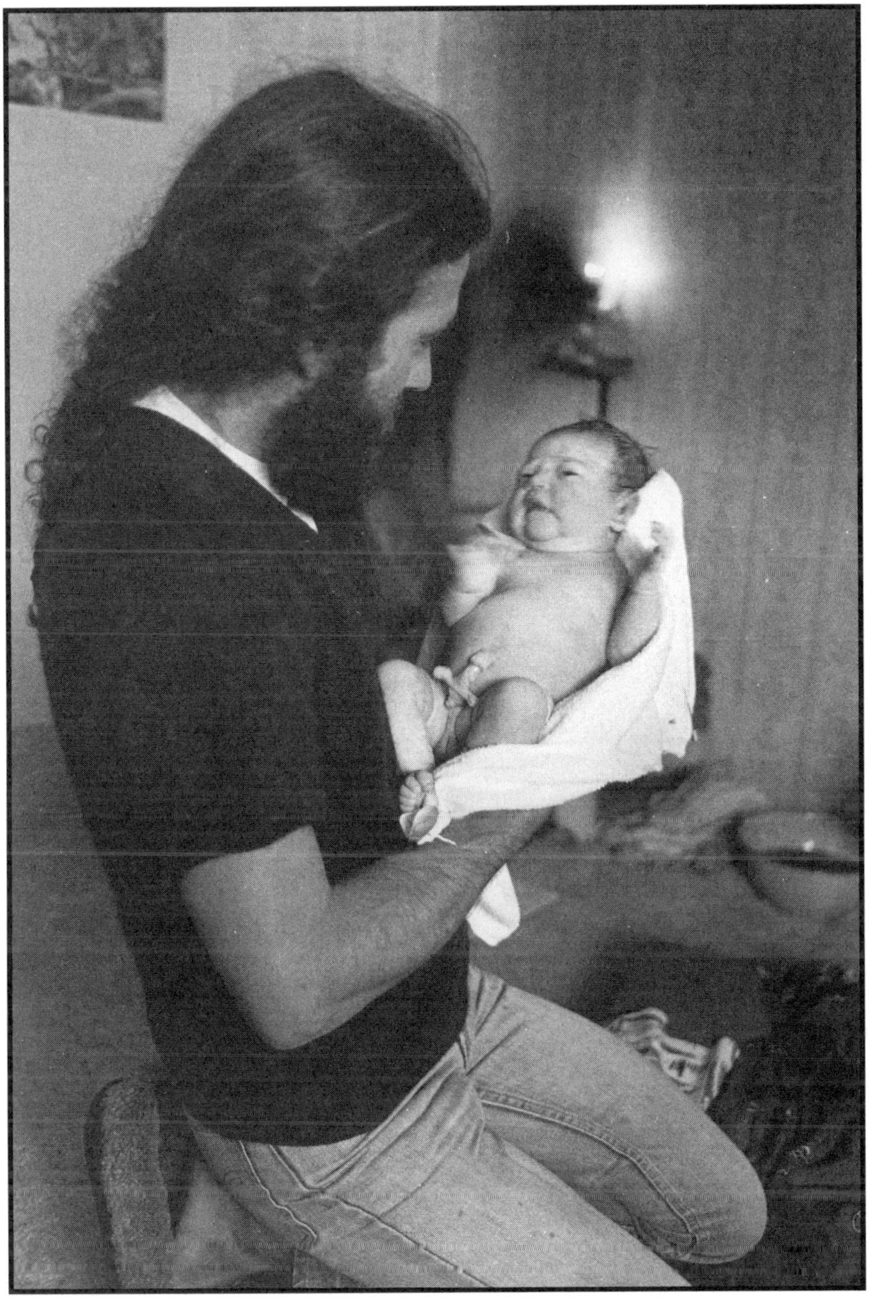

DIFFICULT SITUATIONS

> 'Home birth was much better for me after the previous hospital experience. Then I was harassed by the doctors and nurses who told me to stay put because there was nothing for me to do.'
>
> TONY, FATHER

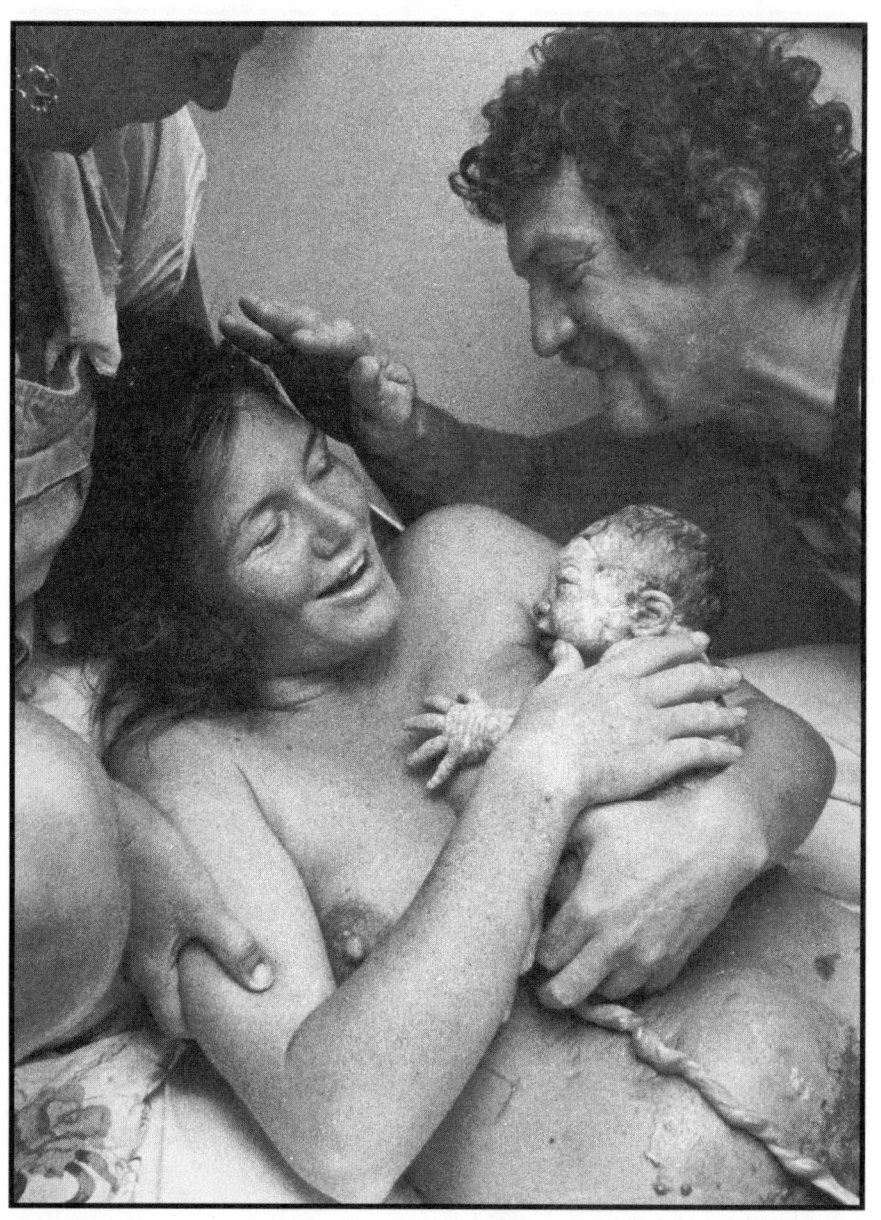

*It was wonderful to be able to share something
so amazing with someone you love. Exciting!
A special bond was formed the moment we three were one.
Holding each other and Baby still joined with Mum. Wow!
The greatest time of my life. To miss that would be
like missing your own birth and never to have lived.*

PETE, FATHER